Nutrition in Nursing: The New Approach

A HANDBOOK OF NURSING SCIENCE

Keats titles of related interest

The Healing Nutrients Within
by Eric Braverman, M.D. with Carl C. Pfeiffer, M.D., Ph.D.

Medical Applications of Clinical Nutrition
Jeffrey Bland, Ph.D., ed.

Mental and Elemental Nutrients
by Carl C. Pfeiffer, M.D., Ph.D.

Nutrition Desk Reference
by Robert H. Garrison, Jr. M.A., R. Ph. and Elizabeth Somer, M. A.

1984–1985; The Yearbook of Nutritional Medicine
Jeffrey Bland, Ph.D., ed.

1986: A Year in Nutritional Medicine
Jeffrey Bland, Ph.D., ed.

Books by Betty Kamen, Ph.D. and Si Kamen

Kids Are What They Eat: What Every Parent Needs to Know About Nutrition

In Pursuit of Youth: Everyday Nutrition for Everyone Over 35

Osteoporosis: What Is It, How to Prevent It, How to Stop It

Total Nutrition During Pregnancy: How to Be Sure You and Your Baby Are Eating the Right Stuff

Total Nutrition for the Breast-Feeding Mother

Nutrition in Nursing: The New Approach

A HANDBOOK OF NURSING SCIENCE

Betty Kamen, Ph.D. and
E. Lynn Fraley, R.N., Dr.P.H.

KEATS PUBLISHING, INC. NEW CANAAN, CONNECTICUT

All of the facts in this book have been very carefully researched, and have been drawn from the scientific literature. However, in no way are any of the suggestions meant to take the place of advice given by physicians.

Library of Congress Cataloging-in-Publication Data

Kamen, Betty.
   Nutrition in nursing.

   Includes bibliographies and index.
   1. Nutrition. 2. Diet therapy. 3. Nursing.
I. Fraley, E. Lynn. II. Title. [DNLM: 1. Nutrition—handbooks. Nutrition—nurses' instruction.
WY 39 K15N]
RM216.K28   1986   613.2′024613   86-27292
ISBN 0-87983-387-4

Nutrition in Nursing: The New Approach
A HANDBOOK OF NURSING SCIENCE
Copyright © 1987 by Betty Kamen, Ph. D. and E. Lynn Fraley, R. N., Dr. P. H.
All Rights Reserved
Printed in the United States of America
Keats Publishing, Inc., 27 Pine Street, New Canaan, Connecticut

Dedicated to Kathleen Anello, R.N.,
who sparked the fuse that led to the enhanced
health and wellbeing of the Kamen family, and
to those who are active in the effort to allow
freedom of choice in health care

The doctors worry that nurses are trying to move away from their historical responsibilities to medicine (meaning, really, to the doctor's orders). The nurses assert that they are their own profession, responsible for their own standards, coequal colleagues with physicians, and they do not wish to become mere ward administrators or technicians.
            LEWIS THOMAS, M.D.
            The Youngest Science
            (New York: Viking, 1983)

CONTENTS

Dedication, v
Acknowledgments, ix
Introduction, xi

1	How Nutrients Work	1
2	Patient Assessment	45
3	Nutrition Versus Calories Versus Absorption	61
4	Nutrient and Drug Interactions	77
5	Nutrient Supplementation	91
6	Disease and Nutritional Support	105
7	Stress and Nutrition	130
8	Politics and Patient Counseling	149
9	Living What You're Teaching	165

Epilogue, 203
Nutrition Education, 206
Index, 208

ACKNOWLEDGMENTS

Thanks to

Robin McAdams, Lisa Morraro, and Susie Shattuck, caregivers at Marin General Hospital, Greenbrae, California

Julie Kahl and Kathie Renick, researchers at Marin General Hospital, Greenbrae, California

Paul Kamen, who, with the help of Norton Utilities, retrieved the lost chapters

Si Kamen and Kenneth Q. Lindahl, Jr., for love and support

INTRODUCTION

When did you decide to become a nurse? If it was when you were a child, do you remember the idealism that pervaded those early hopes and dreams—the plans to soften pain, to ease discomfort and best of all, to help people get well?

Are you disturbed by the popularity of books which relate some shocking facts about hospitals, and advise people about how to stay out of them? (Norman Cousins wrote in his bestselling book that it wasn't until he checked out of the hospital and into a hotel that he began to get well!) And what about cartoons that depict nurses as incompetent or sexy—waking patients to take their sleeping pills, ignoring the call-for-help buzzers while chatting noisily in the hallway or entering the profession just to find husbands?

Can today's health care change for the better? How can nurses initiate this change and help their patients get well? Could nutrition make the difference between good and bad health care in hospitals?

We've asked a lot of questions. We hope that *Nutrition in Nursing* will supply the answers. Reading this book may in fact help you change nursing history.

1

HOW NUTRIENTS WORK

Nutrition cannot be dismissed by vague references to "balanced diets"; it must become a major theme of scientific exploration.
ROGER WILLIAMS

Our knowledge of nutrients is becoming more and more sophisticated. We know, for example, that the need for choline hinges on the availability of methionine, that methionine requirements are lessened when cystine is abundantly supplied and that phenylalanine is decreased if tyrosine is supplied. Complex? Sure it is. That is why computing how much of this or that type of food you should eat to meet a single nutrient requirement doesn't work: *there are too many variables.*

This doesn't mean that you need a Ph.D. in biochemistry

2 Nutrition in Nursing: The New Approach

(in addition to your nursing degrees) to help your patients achieve health through nutrition. Although the study of nutrient pathways is complicated, the concept of maintaining good health is simple. Good health flows from good nourishment. Nourishment is not vitamin A or vitamin C or calcium, nor can it be split into parts. You do not eat a single vitamin or mineral. You do, however, eat a carrot, or an orange or a leafy green. Just as every human being is an integral part of a whole, so nourishment is a gestalt—a totality, and only completeness can create wellbeing. Long before nutrients were isolated and identified, humans enjoyed good health. On the other hand, our sophisticated knowledge has not erased disease. Who knows better than you, the nurse, about the sickness and suffering in spite of our high-tech, late twentieth-century society?

Some of us drive our cars without understanding anything about pistons or clutches or transmissions. We can be healthy without knowledge of polypeptide chains or serotonin catalysts or methyl donors. As a professional, however, you should be familiar with the basic concepts of nutrition. You may already know more *details* than we will explain in this chapter, but without placing the particulars into *conceptual* perspective, they often have little meaning in the everyday world. Understanding these concepts can help you help your patients.

Overview: vitamins and minerals

The energy that keeps you going is created by burning fuel which you get from your environment (food, water, air).

All higher plants can manufacture whatever vitamins they require, but animals must be supplied with vitamins. Although the vitamin requirements of human beings are not exactly like those of lower animals, there are more similarities than differences. Almost all living things need nearly identical nutrients.

We need nutrients for energy, as well as for the building, repair and operation of the mechanisms involved in deriving this energy. Data on vitamin metabolism and mechanisms of action show that no vitamin fulfills its functions in primary form as it occurs in food. The nutrient must undergo transformations assisted by enzymes, other complex substances and transport processes. Other enzymes and enzyme systems convert the nutrient into an active form.

Once converted, the active vitamin is only useful in cooperation with yet other specific enzymes. Although the human body does not manufacture the primary vitamin, it does have to support the final chemical stages before that vitamin can fulfill its mission. These stages in vitamin metabolism are necessary for the realization of the vitamin's functions. Because of these interdependent processes, any disorder in the chain of absorption, transport and activation of a nutrient could result in its failure to be serviceable—even though the vitamin is present in the diet.

Vitamins act as catalysts by assisting other chemical reactions without actually taking part in the process. Their function is not unlike that of the K-pad you use to warm a patient's back. The K-pad provides heat and comfort and may relax muscles, but does not become part of the muscle. Also, since catalysts are not used up in the reactions they promote, only small amounts of them are needed. That is why we require only small amounts of many nutrients.

Here is a specific example of nutrient pathways: animal

cells obtain much of the energy required for life through oxidation of the carbohydrate, glucose. This takes place in many intermediate steps; energy is set free very gradually instead of all at once. Several of the B-complex vitamins have been found in enzymes and coenzymes, each of which catalyzes only one special step in the oxidation of the carbohydrate. The absence of any one of these enzymes signals a failure of some indispensable link in the chain of tissue oxidations. *The lack of a vitamin that is an essential part of such an enzyme can cripple vital oxidation processes in cells.* As a consequence, tissues all over the body may suffer. This is not unlike the old legend, "For want of a horseshoe nail the war was lost."

The cell is the center of this activity. To achieve and maintain optimum health, the cell must be adequately nourished. Unfortunately, cells do not automatically receive all of the nutritional elements they require. Again, knowledge of the maze-like characteristics of nutritional biochemistry is not essential for the care of your patients. What is essential, however, is knowledge of nutrients, because nutrients work as a team. Only with team effort can the cell function with optimal efficiency.

The cooperation and the extraordinary interdependence of *all* nutrients complicate their classification. Categories are not as helpful as previously believed. Nonetheless, the categories are widely used, and you should be familiar with them.

WATER-SOLUBLE VITAMINS

Water-soluble vitamins—the B vitamins and vitamin C—are not usually stored in the body (except for vitamin B12 and a few complex phenomena). For the most part, there are daily losses of these nutrients through normal metabolism, thus dictating their frequent replenishment. The B vitamins are thiamin (B1), riboflavin (B2), niacin (B3), pantothenic acid (B5), pyridoxine (B6), cobalamin (B12), folic acid, choline, inositol, para-aminobenzoic acid (PABA) and biotin.

The B vitamins are widely distributed in meats and vegetables, but no single food contains the full range in sufficient quantities to meet your needs. The B vitamins are found in yeast, fruit, vegetables, nuts, meat and fish. Because they are water-soluble, they go down the drain with the water in which they've been cooked; and because they are located in the outer husk of seeds and cereals, processed foods, such as bleached flour and polished rice, completely lack them.

The best sources of vitamin C are citrus fruits. But citrus is high on the allergy list (see Chapter 6), so other foods might be preferable for daily vitamin C rations. Apples, blueberries, brussels sprouts, cabbage, cantaloupe, carrots, celery, chard, endive, peas, peppers, pineapple, rhubarb, spinach, tomatoes, turnip greens and watercress all contain vitamin C.

Most water-soluble vitamins are components of enzyme systems. This means they initiate important metabolic events.

FAT-SOLUBLE VITAMINS

Fat-soluble vitamins—A, D, E and K—are stored in the body, relieving us of the responsibility of acquiring them on a day-to-day basis—except where need is extreme. These vitamins are found in foods in association with fats, and are absorbed along with fats in the diet. Conditions unfavorable to normal fat uptake impair their absorption. Good sources of fat are primal foods like eggs, nuts, avocados, seeds, fish and some vegetables. Proper absorption is disturbed by consuming processed oils (especially rancid salad dressings), hydrogenated fats and fats which have been repeatedly heated at high temperatures.

Fat-soluble vitamins participate in cell differentiation and growth. Their general function is to regulate the manufacture of protein.

Vitamins differ from the mineral elements in that they are organic substances, while they differ from hormones because (at least for the most part) they are not formed within the body but *must be supplied in food.*

MINERALS

Minerals, some of which are called trace elements because they occur in small quantities, are both interrelated and balanced against each other, like members of teams in a tug-of-war. A single mineral doesn't work by itself. Knowing the quantity of one mineral in an individual's diet has little significance without knowing the quantities of other minerals. Diagnostic interpretation using the amount of a single mineral is like one hand clapping.

The body needs at least thirteen different minerals, which must be derived from the diet. Whole grains, nuts and seeds, and leafy greens are good sources of minerals, which include potassium, calcium, magnesium, manganese and zinc.

It cannot be emphasized enough that the requirement for a specific nutrient is contingent on the presence of other nutrients. Unlike drugs, single nutrients do not function to block or accelerate metabolic activity with immediacy. Years ago we associated poor vision with lack of vitamin A, and we believed we could improve bone health with calcium. Now we know that no amount of vitamin A without zinc (and other nutrients) can improve eyesight, just as calcium intake will never repair bones without magnesium and vitamin D (and other nutrients). Synergism is the name of the game. And even that is an oversimplification because it doesn't address the antagonistic effects of other substances. A deficiency or overabundance of a single nutrient results in a disruption of the concatenation.

Nutrient utilization

Although some of today's guidelines for good health have been known for millennia, the existence of specific nutrients was not recognized until this century. The quantities of these substances present in foods were too small to have been detected by chemists. It took many years before scientists realized that diseases might be caused by the *lack* of something in the diet. Now, doctors commonly diagnose subclinical deficiencies of certain nutrients. This new knowledge has caused us to come full cycle; we now add to foods some of the nutrients that were removed during processing.

Whether food is taken directly from plants or indirectly from animals, the plant cell is ultimately the source of the nutrients required for health. Green leaves are heavily endowed with nutrients, formed from simple substances (CO_2 and H_2O) with the aid of sunlight. Green, growing shoots of plants also have a high nutrient content, as do seeds and grains. Fruits, root vegetables and vegetables with a high water content usually have a lower quantity of most nutrients, although there are exceptions. Nutrient content may vary depending on the soil in which the foods are grown,

8   Nutrition in Nursing: The New Approach

their stage of ripeness when picked, conditions of storage, length of storage and processing. Animals obtain most of their nutrients either directly from plants or indirectly from animals which have fed on plants. (Many animals can form a few vitamins in their own bodies—vitamins which humans can only acquire from food. Vitamin C is one such vitamin.)

It is easier to describe the effects of nutrients or the lack of them in food than to define them as a group, because they differ widely in their chemical nature and in their physiological action. We thus encourage you to read and study the details of the Nutrient Chart. It provides a clear picture of vitamin and mineral functions, food sources, RDAs, allies, antagonists, deficiency symptoms and special needs. A general idea of the contents of this chart will serve as an excellent reference tool.

The chart has been compiled from a variety of current references. Most foods contain almost all nutrients, but the foods listed below are those in which the nutrient designated can be found in significant quantities. Eating any food in its natural or "primal" form offers the greatest nutrient supply.

The *Recommended Daily Allowances* (RDAs) may be regarded as the minimum amount of a nutrient that an individual requires each day. RDAs are often barely higher than the least amount necessary to protect against deficiency-related diseases (See Chapter 5). The optimal dosage varies from person to person.

We have intentionally eliminated those food products which we regard as unhealthful.

Nutrient chart—vitamins

VITAMIN A

FUNCTION
Maintains integrity of mucous membranes; fights infections, allergies, air pollutants; required for growth and repair of cells, important for eyes, skin, hair, teeth, ears, bony structures, synthesis of RNA and reproductive system; necessary for protein metabolism; protects night vision; aids in detoxification; antioxidant; protects against cancer

SOURCES
Preformed: liver, fish liver oils, kidney, eggs, dairy products
Provitamin: carrots, apricots, broccoli, cantaloupe, parsley and other leafy greens, turnips and other yellow vegetables

RDA
Adults: 5000 IU; children: 2500 IU

ALLIES
B-complex, vitamins D, E and C

ANTAGONISTS
Air pollutants, glare or strong light, nitrate fertilizers, mineral oil, high temperatures, oil, vitamin D deficiency, alcohol, coffee, cortisone

DEFICIENCY CAN CAUSE
Poor growth, major anemias, spinal cord degeneration, night blindness, blindness, dry skin, faulty tooth development, gas-

trointestinal (G.I.) disorders, inflamed tongue, disturbed metabolism, allergies, appetite loss, itching/burning eyes, loss of taste and smell, eye styes

NEED INCREASED WITH
Diabetes, use of oral contraceptives, aging, stress, pregnancy, acne, alcoholism, arthritis, bronchitis, cystitis

VITAMIN D

FUNCTION
Helps calcium absorption, essential for normal bones and teeth; necessary for utilization of calcium and phosphorus; helps maintain normal kidney function, heart action, nervous system, and blood clotting

SOURCES
Sunshine, liver, fish liver oils, eggs, brewer's yeast, shrimp, salmon, tuna, avocados, fortified milk

RDA
400 IU

ALLIES
B-complex, vitamins A and C, calcium

ANTAGONISTS
Cortisone, anticonvulsants, diphenhydantoin, inadequate exposure to sunlight, liver disease, mineral oil, laxatives, aflatoxins, antacids

DEFICIENCY CAN CAUSE
Skeletal malformation, rickets, osteoporosis, tooth problems, reduced parathyroid activity, diminished kidney function, diminished muscle tone, insomnia, fluoride toxicity

NEED INCREASED WITH
Pregnancy, aging, heavy metal toxicity, lack of sunlight, lactation

VITAMIN E

FUNCTION
Antioxidant; essential for the maintenance of red blood cells, circulatory, nervous, digestive, excretory and respiratory systems, reproduction; maintains integrity of cell membranes; protects against air pollutants and other free radicals, thereby retarding aging and wrinkles; promotes ability to respond to stress; protects essential fatty acids; aids in preventing lung disease

SOURCES
Whole grains, eggs, molasses, avocados, sweet potatoes, leafy greens, cold-pressed vegetable oils, asparagus, broccoli, cabbage, yeast, meat, nuts, organ meats

RDA
Men: 15 IU; women: 12 IU; children: 10 IU

ALLIES
Vitamins A and C, B-complex, selenium, manganese

12 Nutrition in Nursing: The New Approach

ANTAGONISTS
Oxidizing agents, food processing, rancid fats and oils, inorganic iron, the Pill, mineral oil, chlorine, thyroid hormone

DEFICIENCY CAN CAUSE
Clinical deficiency diseases just being recognized; anemia, reproductive, muscular or cardiovascular problems, and intermittent claudication

NEED INCREASED WITH
Increased polyunsaturated fat intake, pregnancy and lactation, air pollution, stress; burns; menopause, benign breast tumors, heart conditions and arteriosclerosis

VITAMIN K

FUNCTION
Vital to blood clotting; liver coenzyme required for energy metabolism and respiration (fat-soluble); implicated in electron transport

SOURCES
Leafy greens, eggs, alfalfa, soy bean oil, pork liver, cauliflower, cabbage, intestinal flora

RDA
Not established; optimum: 300 to 500 mcg

ALLIES
Vitamins A, C and E

ANTAGONISTS
Anticoagulants, antibiotics, sulfonamides, mineral oil, aspirin and aspirin substitutes, radiation, rancid fats, X-rays

DEFICIENCY CAN CAUSE
Prolonged blood coagulation time, increased incidence of hemorrhage (rare), hemorrhage in newborn; diarrhea, miscarriages

NEED INCREASED WITH
Infancy, surgery, major medical problems, certain medications, aging, anticoagulants, celiac disease, women in labor

VITAMIN C

FUNCTION
Important for cell, tissue, nervous system, tooth and bone formation and repair; aids in formation and maintenance of capillary walls; healing wounds and burns; antioxidant; works against causes of aging; regulates amino acid metabolism; maintains connective tissues (water-soluble); potentiates iron absorption and some hormone manufacture; antihistamine effect

SOURCES
Citrus, acerola berries and rose hips, berries, cantaloupes, tomatoes, potatoes, papaya, parsley, peppers, cabbage, green vegetables (raw or minimally cooked), black currants

RDA
Adults: 60 mg; children: 40 mg

14 Nutrition in Nursing: The New Approach

ALLIES
Bioflavonoids, B-complex, vitamins A, K and E, testosterone, hormones

ANTAGONISTS
Air pollution, industrial toxins, smoking, alcohol, aspirin, anticoagulants, antidepressants, diuretics, antibiotics, high fever, copper, exposure to air and heat, storage and processing, cortisone, the Pill

DEFICIENCY CAN CAUSE
Scurvy, bacterial infection, cell deterioration, bruising, edema, hemorrhaging, tooth and gum problems, anemia, lethargy, poor digestion

NEED INCREASED WITH
Stress, pregnancy and lactation, viral and bacterial infections, smoking, aging, burns, dialysis, certain medications (sometimes accelerating detoxification; other times potentiating medicine's effect)

BIOFLAVONOIDS

FUNCTION
Strengthen artery walls; maintain blood capillaries; help prevent viral, bacterial and fungal infections; antioxidant; helpful in herpes and certain diabetic cataracts; anti-inflammatory

SOURCES
Citrus pulp, red peppers, tomatoes, apricots, rhubarb, buckwheat, onions with colored skins, grapes, black currants, cherries, cantaloupe, rose hips

RDA
Not established; optimum: 25 mg

ALLIES
Vitamin C

ANTAGONISTS
Air pollution, industrial toxins, smoking, alcohol, anticoagulants

DEFICIENCY CAN CAUSE
Edema, spontaneous hemorrhaging, easy bruising, inflammation of mucous membranes

NEED INCREASED WITH
Smoking, menstruation, bruising, hemorrhoids, varicose veins, reproduction, aging, cardiovascular disease

THIAMIN (Vitamin B1)

FUNCTION
Antioxidant; required for cellular synthesis of acetylcholine; helps maintain health of nerves, heart muscle and digestive tissue; promotes cellular growth and repair; helps create food energy; aids digestion; necessary for carbohydrate metabolism

SOURCES
Brewer's yeast, organ meats, whole grains, fish, fruits, eggs, milk, legumes, sunflower seeds, nuts (especially almonds), green vegetables

RDA
Adults: 1.4 mg; children: 0.7 mg

16 Nutrition in Nursing: The New Approach

ALLIES
Other B-complex vitamins, and vitamins C and E

ANTAGONISTS
Physical and emotional stress, food additives (particularly nitrites and sulfites), baking soda, air pollution, alcohol, carbohydrates, antibiotics, overcooking, coffee, fever, excessive sugar, tobacco, high temperatures, milling of grains, food preparation (especially of beans and baked goods)

DEFICIENCY CAN CAUSE
Loss of appetite, insomnia, irritability, impairment of cardiovascular system, nervous and gastrointestinal systems, fatigue, weakness, weight loss, poor reflexes, memory loss, edema, shortness of breath, beriberi

NEED INCREASED WITH
Pregnancy, lactation, increased carbohydrates in diet, alcoholism, aging, surgery, fever, cardiac problems, allergy

RIBOFLAVIN (Vitamin B2)

FUNCTION
Assists in metabolism of carbohydrates, fats and proteins; aids nervous system and wound healing; necessary in energy release; helps regulate hormones and growth and development of fetus

SOURCES
Organ and other meats, milk, fish, brewer's yeast, eggs, leafy greens, broccoli, yogurt, whole grains, legumes, intestinal bacterial flora

RDA
Adults: 1.7 mg; children: 0.8 mg

ALLIES
Other B-complex vitamins, protein, vitamins E and A

ANTAGONISTS
Antibiotics, the Pill, exposure to light, azo dyes

DEFICIENCY CAN CAUSE
Lesions of lips, mouth, eyes, skin, and genitals; fatigue; loss of appetite; severe personality disturbances, anxiety, digestive upset, hypertension, cataracts, acne, anemia, photophobia, seborrheic dermatitis at nose, magenta tongue

NEED INCREASED WITH
Pregnancy, old age, increased protein in diet, liver damage, dialysis

NIACIN (Vitamin B3)

FUNCTION
Converts food to energy; aids nervous system; antischizophrenia agent; necessary for metabolism of fats, protein, and carbohydrates; regulates hormones and many enzymatic reactions; helps cellular respiration and wound healing; acts as a vasodilator

SOURCES
Liver, lean meat, poultry, tuna, halibut, legumes, whole grains, butter, yeast, nuts

RDA
Adults: 18 mg; children: 9 mg

ALLIES
Other B-complex vitamins, vitamins A, C and D, phosphorus, tryptophan with B6

ANTAGONISTS
Alcohol, physical and emotional stress, dietary carbohydrates, antibiotics, coffee, high-corn diets, tuberculosis treatment

DEFICIENCY CAN CAUSE
Pellagra, dermatitis, gastrointestinal and central nervous system disturbances, diarrhea, irritability, headache, memory loss, loss of appetite, insomnia, red and painful tongue

NEED INCREASED WITH
Alcoholism, old age, associated B6 deficiency, angina pectoris, poor circulation

PANTOTHENIC ACID (Vitamin B5)

FUNCTION
Contributes to metabolism of carbohydrates, fat and protein; important for cellular metabolism and for synthesis of essential body fats, including cholesterol; of great importance in dealing with stress and adrenal function; necessary for synthesis of antibodies; antioxidant; helps formation of hemoglobin

SOURCES
Beef liver and other organ meats, eggs, nuts, legumes, whole grains, broccoli, cauliflower, cabbage

How Nutrients Work

RDA
Adults: 10 mg; children: 5 mg

ALLIES
Other B-complex vitamins, vitamins A, C and E, calcium

ANTAGONISTS
Methyl bromide (insecticide fumigant used for storing foods), stress, alcohol, coffee, dry heat, acid or alkaline medium, high-temperature frying, frozen meat

DEFICIENCY CAN CAUSE
Increased susceptibility to infection, loss of appetite, depression, constipation, neuromotor disorders, fatigue, sleep disorders, eczema, hair loss, cramps, hypoglycemia, apathy, abdominal pain, tingling hands or feet, muscle cramps, impaired coordination, loss of antibody production, impaired adrenal function

NEED INCREASED WITH
Postoperative shock, wounds or infection, cirrhosis, marginal diabetes, physical and emotional stress, aging, hypoglycemia, cystitis, arthritis, pregnancy and lactation (important because vitamin B5 levels are usually lower in pregnancy and lactation)

PYRIDOXINE (Vitamin B6)

FUNCTION
Necessary for synthesis of protein and antibodies; important for red blood cells, nervous system, and healthy skin; essential to healthy teeth and gums; regulates body fluids and almost all enzymatic reactions; glycogen-energy release

SOURCES
Liver, poultry, kidney, whole grains, fish (especially herring and salmon), eggs, lean meat, yeast, soybeans, walnuts, cantaloupe, leafy greens, bananas, prunes, raisins

RDA
Adults: 2 mg; children: 0.6 mg

ALLIES
Other B-complex vitamins, vitamin C, magnesium, potassium, linoleic acid, unsaturated fatty acids

ANTAGONISTS
Penicillamine, hydrazide drugs, L-dopa, isoniazid, cortisone, the Pill, high-protein diet, marijuana, milling of grains, high temperatures, food processing, tuberculosis drugs, light, alkalis

DEFICIENCY CAN CAUSE
Anemia, lymphopenia (white blood cell disorder), neuronal disorders including convulsions, neuritis, depression, kidney stones, dermatitis of eyes, nose, mouth, back of ears, edema

NEED INCREASED WITH
Pregnancy, lactation, increased fat or protein in diet, low hemoglobin, nerve development or growth in infancy, the Pill, aging, Parkinson's disease

COBALAMIN (vitamin B12)

FUNCTION
Necessary for proper function of bone marrow, nervous sys-

tem, myelin formation, gastrointestinal tract, and red blood cells; prevents certain forms of anemia; assists in synthesis of nucleic acids (RNA, DNA); important for carbohydrate metabolism and normal blood ascorbic levels

SOURCES
Liver, kidney, fish, shellfish (especially crab and oysters), algae, tempeh, intestinal bacterial flora (*note*: intestinal flora are important because their presence indicates that the body manufactures its own supply of the nutrient, given the right environment in the intestine)

RDA
Adults: 3 mcg; children: 3 mcg

ALLIES
Other B-complex vitamins, vitamins A, C and E, choline, inositol, potassium, calcium

ANTAGONISTS
Aspirin and its substitutes, codeine, the Pill, alcohol, heat (especially severe heating of meat), and nitrous oxide (nitrous oxide is used frequently in dentists' offices)

DEFICIENCY CAN CAUSE
Pernicious anemia, poor growth, disrupted carbohydrate metabolism, memory loss, paranoia, nervous disorders, ataxia (interference with bodily movements)

NEED INCREASED WITH
Vegetarianism, the Pill, inadequate absorption of vitamin B12 (requires sublingual or IV supplementation), surgery, epilepsy, liver disease, dialysis, ileitis, sprue, eye problems, tapeworm

FOLIC ACID

FUNCTION
Works with B12 in production of red blood cells; aids metabolism and development of nerve cells; maintains nervous system, gastrointestinal tract and white blood cells; helps skin; acts as antidepressant; involved in production of choline and methionine; essential for nucleic acid production; regulates fetal development; involved in cell division

SOURCES
Leafy greens, asparagus, whole grains, nuts, legumes, yeast, liver, kidney, tuna, broccoli, oranges, intestinal bacterial flora

RDA
Adults: 400 mcg; children: 200 mcg

ALLIES
Other B-complex vitamins, vitamin C, estradiol, testosterone

ANTAGONISTS
Alcohol, physical and emotional stress, the Pill, sulfonamides, aspirin, anticonvulsant drugs, air, light, moderate heat, processing, storage

DEFICIENCY CAN CAUSE
Certain anemias, inflamed tongue, depression, nervousness, cell and tissue disruptions, premature gray hair, hair loss

NEED INCREASED WITH
Pregnancy and lactation, cancer, blood disorders, intestinal problems, the Pill, depression, low white cell count, anemia, psoriasis, sprue, sickle cell disease

BIOTIN

FUNCTION
Necessary for intermediate metabolism of fats, carbohydrates and proteins; maintains bone, bone marrow, sweat glands, skin, nerve tissue, blood cells, and hair color

SOURCES
Liver and other organ meats, brewer's yeast, mushrooms, nuts, corn, eggs, legumes, cauliflower, intestinal bacterial flora

RDA
Not established; optimum: 100 to 300 mcg

ALLIES
Other B-complex vitamins, vitamins A and D, testosterone, manganese

ANTAGONISTS
Raw egg white (avidin), choline, antibiotics, sulfonamides, alcohol, coffee, processed food

DEFICIENCY CAN CAUSE
Mild skin disorders, lassitude, anorexia, anemia, muscle pain, nausea, depression, high cholesterol, insomnia, hair loss, conjunctivitis

NEED INCREASED WITH
Genetic impairment, antibiotics, dry hair, consumption of large quantities of raw egg white

INOSITOL

FUNCTION
Involved in reactions controlling metabolism of fats; necessary to brain metabolism; lowers cholesterol; regulates oil glands and hair growth

SOURCES
Whole grains, brewer's yeast, lecithin, nuts, seeds, liver, beef brain and heart, vegetables

RDA
Not established; optimum: 75 to 2000 mg

ALLIES
Choline, biotin, vitamin E

ANTAGONISTS
Antibiotics, mineral oil, diarrhea, high cholesterol levels, pesticides, water, food processing, alcohol, caffeine

DEFICIENCY CAN CAUSE
Hardening of arteries, fatty degeneration of liver; may be related to nerve damage of muscular dystrophy and hair loss

NEED INCREASED WITH
Toxic chemical exposure, heart conditions, heavy caffeine use

PABA (Para-aminobenzoic acid)

FUNCTION
Aids in utilization of proteins and in formation of red blood cells when used topically; regulates oil glands; blocks sun; offers free radical protection

SOURCES
Brewer's yeast, whole grains, yogurt, meat (especially liver and other organs), seeds, nuts, leafy greens

RDA
Not established; optimum: 30 to 75 mg

ALLIES
Pantothenic acid, folic acid, vitamin C

ANTAGONISTS
Estrogen, sulfonamides, water, food processing, alcohol

DEFICIENCY CAN CAUSE
Some anemias, skin disorders

NEED INCREASED WITH
High-protein diet, ozone toxicity, burns, excessive sun exposure (applied topically), vitiligo and other skin conditions

CHOLINE

FUNCTION
Required for transmission of nerve impulses, synthesis of acetylcholine, fatty acid metabolism; helpful in preventing arteriosclerosis

SOURCES
Lecithin, egg yolk, liver, legumes, green leafy vegetables, brewer's yeast, brains, whole grains

RDA
Not established; optimum varies

ALLIES
Other B-complex vitamins (especially choline), methionine

ANTAGONISTS
Water, food processing, alcohol, sulfa drugs

DEFICIENCY CAN CAUSE
Chronic hepatic disease, cirrhosis, liver steatosis, stomach ulcers, high blood pressure, loss of memory, anemia, heart and circulatory disease, muscle weakness

NEED INCREASED WITH
Neurological disorders, especially Alzheimer's disease, high cholesterol levels, toxic exposures, weak or thin nails, pregnancy and lactation, hardening of arteries, alcoholism, circulatory problems

Nutrient chart—minerals

CALCIUM

FUNCTION
Builds bones and teeth; buffer for acid/alkaline balance; regulates certain body processes; aids blood clotting; regulates

heart rhythm; contributes to vitality, endurance and relaxation; helpful in utilization of iron

SOURCES
Yogurt, acidophilus, shellfish, egg yolk, sardines and salmon (with bones), soybeans, tofu, green vegetables (turnips and mustard), broccoli, kale, bone marrow, bone

RDA
Adults: 1200 mg; pregnant women: 1600 mg; children: 1000 mg; under age 4: 800 mg; under 1 year: 600 mg

ALLIES
Vitamins D, A, C and E, magnesium, phosphorus, iron, hydrochloric acid (HCL), manganese, mild physical activity

ANTAGONISTS
High phosphorus, high-protein diet, stress, inactivity, excessive physical activity; magnesium, vitamin D and HCL deficiencies; cortisone, aluminum, antacids, laxatives, diuretics, aging, anticonvulsants

DEFICIENCIES CAN CAUSE
Osteoarthritis, osteoporosis, pyorrhea, tooth problems, heart palpitations, menstrual cramps, hypertension, insomnia, muscle cramps

NEED INCREASED WITH
Lactation; postmenopause; eating meat; smoking

MAGNESIUM

FUNCTION
Necessary for normal function of brain and spinal cord, enzyme energy conversions, calcium and vitamin C metabolism; vital to carbohydrate metabolism; important for neuromuscular contractions and bone and tooth enamel

SOURCES
Soy, nuts, whole grains, legumes, green leafy vegetables, molasses, seaweed, seeds

RDA
Adults: 300 mg; pregnant and lactating women: 450 mg

ALLIES
Calcium, phosphorus, protein, vitamins D, C and E, B-complex vitamins, sodium, potassium

ANTAGONISTS
Diuretics, high cholesterol levels, large intake of calcium and phosphorus, barbiturates

DEFICIENCIES CAN CAUSE
Dental problems, bone problems, muscle tension, increased heart rate, exhaustion, kidney stones, convulsions, dizziness, hearing disorders

NEED INCREASED WITH
Pregnancy, chronic alcoholism, atherosclerosis, arterial edema, recurrent spontaneous abortion, low-birth-weight infants, anxiety

PHOSPHORUS

FUNCTION
Has more functions than any other mineral element; works with calcium and vitamin D to give strength and rigidity to bones and teeth; important in nerve function; essential in all cell metabolism, cell repair and muscle contractions; part of DNA molecule

SOURCES
Yogurt, poultry, fish, meat, cheese, nuts, cereals, legumes, brewer's yeast

RDA
Men: 800 mg; women: 1200 mg; children: 240 to 1200 mg

ALLIES
Calcium, iron, protein, vitamin D, hydrochloric acid

ANTAGONISTS
Magnesium, iron, sugar, fats, aluminum, antacids

DEFICIENCIES CAN CAUSE
Bone and teeth problems, fatigue, nervousness, loss of appetite, overweight (deficiencies are uncommon, however)

NEED INCREASED WITH
Sepsis, Reye's syndrome

POTASSIUM

FUNCTION
Works with sodium to maintain body fluids; involved in nervous and muscular systems; necessary for normal muscle tone, nerves, heart action, enzyme reactions, fluid balance, glucose absorption and growth

SOURCES
Bananas, oranges, fruit, meat, fish, poultry, cereals, vegetables, seaweed, nuts, seeds, legumes, dried fruit, blackstrap molasses

RDA
Not established, but estimated to range from 2000 to 6000 mg daily

ALLIES
Vitamin B6, sodium

ANTAGONISTS
Cortisone, caffeine, stress, alcohol, laxatives, diuretics, sugar, salt, high cholesterol levels, diarrhea, excessive sweating, aldosterone, colchicine (drug for gout)

DEFICIENCIES CAN CAUSE
Edema, high blood pressure, nervousness, depressed heartbeat, insomnia, constipation, impaired glucose metabolism, general weakness, poor reflexes, acne

NEED INCREASED WITH
Heavy physical exertion, sweating, diarrhea, excessive vomiting, hypertension

SODIUM

FUNCTION
Maintains normal fluid levels in cell; determines osmotic pressure of fluids outside cell; helps in acid/alkaline balance; necessary for muscle contractions

SOURCES
Seafoods, meats, poultry, green vegetables, cheese, soft water, processed foods, kelp, smoked meats

RDA
Dependent on body losses; average estimated to be 3 grams of sodium chloride

ALLIES
Potassium, vitamin B6

ANTAGONISTS
Hot weather, dehydration, diuretics

DEFICIENCIES CAN CAUSE
Alkalosis, muscle cramps, nausea, edema, high blood pressure, irritability, intestinal gas, weight loss, impaired conversion of carbohydrates into fats, lassitude, aches in skeletal muscles (deficiencies are uncommon, however)

NEED INCREASED WITH
Diarrhea, vomiting, fever, any fluid loss, intense perspiration, adrenal cortical insufficiency

IRON

FUNCTION
Required in manufacture of hemoglobin, helps carry oxygen in blood, important in protein metabolism, bone growth, disease resistance, and in preventing fatigue

SOURCES
Liver, meat, legumes, whole grains, potatoes, eggs, leafy greens, dried fruit, seaweed, nuts, cherries

RDA
Men: 10 to 18 mg; women: 18 mg; children: 10 to 18 mg

ALLIES
Vitamins C, E, B6, and B12, folic acid, copper, phosphorus, calcium, nickel, cobalt

ANTAGONISTS
Zinc, excess phosphorus, bleeding, coffee and tea, intestinal parasites, lack of HCL, antacids (bicarbonate), oxalates, tetracycline

DEFICIENCIES CAN CAUSE
Anemia, weakness, fatigue, headache, palpitation, heartburn

NEED INCREASED WITH
Pregnancy, lactation, aging, nosebleeds (or any blood loss), excessive menstruation, formula feeding of infants, rapid growth

ZINC

FUNCTION
Necessary for normal skeletal growth and repair of body tissues; aids normal tissue function, protein and carbohydrate metabolism; part of enzymes that move carbon dioxide to lungs; important to brain, thyroid, liver, kidney function, hair, skin, prostate and phosphorus metabolism; participates in nucleic acid and protein metabolism; facilitates release of vitamin A stores

SOURCES
Oysters, herring, meat, liver and other organ meats, eggs, milk, bones, brewer's yeast, legumes, nuts, paprika, whole grains, mushrooms, leafy greens

RDA
15 milligrams; pregnant women: 20 mg; lactating women: 25 mg

ALLIES
Copper, calcium, phosphorus, vitamins C and A, certain amino acids (cysteine, methionine, histidine)

ANTAGONISTS
Alcohol, excess calcium, cadmium, unleavened bread, parasites, grain processing, high phytate levels, the Pill

DEFICIENCIES CAN CAUSE
Slow healing, retarded growth, baldness, delayed sexual maturation, retarded mental development, fatigue, decreased alertness, stretch marks in pregnancy, white spots on fingernails, sterility

NEED INCREASED WITH
Wound healing and burns, surgical incisions, poor appetite, decreased smell and taste acuity

COPPER

FUNCTION
Involved in storage of iron to form hemoglobin; necessary to maintain blood cell production, absorption and utilization of iron, and oxidation of vitamin C; contributes to bone formation; helps calm nerves and promote clear thinking; vital to enzyme system; helps form myelin sheath; helps produce RNA

SOURCES
Oysters, liver, nuts, legumes, mushrooms, avocados, leafy greens, seaweed, raisins, blueberries, whole grains, meat, fish

RDA
Adults: 2 to 3 mg; children: 0.5 to 3 mg

ALLIES
Other minerals, provided they are all in balance, including copper

ANTAGONISTS
Excess zinc, calcium, cadmium and iron; competition from excess minerals, phytates, fiber, calcium carbonate and ascorbic acid

DEFICIENCIES CAN CAUSE
Pernicious anemia, respiratory problems, retarded growth, edema and bone demineralization (deficiency is rare, however)

MANGANESE

NEED INCREASED WITH
Infants fed cow's milk; premature infants; intravenous feeding; tropical and nontropical sprue

MANGANESE

FUNCTION
Involved in growth, calcium and phosphorus metabolism, as well as enzyme activation; aids in utilization of vitamins B1 and E; important for brain, pancreas, heart, spleen, bones and lymph; vital to various enzyme systems involved in protein and energy metabolism; essential to central nervous system; helps in synthesis of fatty acids and cholesterol

SOURCES
Nuts, whole grains, legumes, tea, cloves, eggs, carrots, beets, celery, liver, pineapple

RDA
Not established, but estimated amounts are 2.5 to 5 mg

ALLIES
Vitamins B1 and E, calcium, phosphorus

ANTAGONISTS
High calcium/phosphorus ratio, bran, soy beans, food refining, hydralazine (hypotensive drug)

DEFICIENCIES CAN CAUSE
Diabetes, ataxia (lack of muscle coordination), hearing loss, convulsions, glandular disorders, growth retardation, infertility, skeletal disorders, disturbed lipid metabolism, disturbed nervous system

36 Nutrition in Nursing: The New Approach

NEED INCREASED WITH
Lactation and pregnancy, professional athletes, those taking L-dopa

CHROMIUM

FUNCTION
Important in insulin metabolism and glucose conversion; involved in synthesis of fatty acids and cholesterol in liver; associated with RNA

SOURCES
Brewer's yeast, black pepper and other condiments, calf's liver, whole grains, meats, milk, poultry

RDA
0.05 to 2 mg

ALLIES
Protein

ANTAGONISTS
Air pollution, stress, food refining, average American diet (this is the only country with chromium deficiencies)

DEFICIENCIES CAN CAUSE
Diabetes, hypoglycemia, atherosclerosis, retarded growth, high cholesterol levels, aortic plaques, corneal opacification

NEED INCREASED WITH
Low birth weight, glucose metabolism problems (such as diabetes or hypoglycemia), high cholesterol levels, pregnancy and lactation, atherosclerotic heart disease, intravenous feedings

SELENIUM

FUNCTION
Helps maintain liver and muscle function, important for tissue elasticity, antioxidant of fats, contributes to growth and hair; may be protective against cancer and heart disease; used in protein matrix of teeth

SOURCES
Brewer's yeast, organ meats, sea food, whole grains, brown rice, garlic, cabbage, eggs, milk, chicken, broccoli, tomatoes, onions, tuna

RDA
Not established, but estimated needs are 150 to 300 mcg

ALLIES
Vitamin E, protein, sulfate

ANTAGONISTS
Mercury and cadmium

DEFICIENCIES CAN CAUSE
Arteriosclerosis, cancer, kwashiorkor, premature aging, growth retardation, cataract formation, toxicity of oxidants, liver damage

NEED INCREASED WITH
People living in low selenium areas; those exposed to radiation toxicity, toxic-metal poisoning, benzene toxicity and high air pollution; infertility; exposure to chemical carcinogenesis

SILICON

FUNCTION
Important in carbohydrate metabolism and normal connective tissue development; aids in calcium and collagen absorption; keeps skin permeable to liquids; has growth-promoting effects

SOURCES
High-fiber foods, vegetables, water, grains, organ meats, milk, alfalfa

RDA
Not established

ALLIES
Calcium and fiber

ANTAGONISTS
High temperatures and any food processing that deletes or reduces fiber

DEFICIENCIES CAN CAUSE
Deformed bones, slow growth, depressed connective tissue development

NEED INCREASED WITH
Osteoporosis, osteoarthritis; essential for those on purified diets—may be important in space travel

FLUORINE

FUNCTION
Protects teeth during childhood and adolescence; essential for normal growth; reduces skeletal mineral loss

SOURCES
Water supplies (but better obtained through food sources because of toxic risk), seafoods (especially salmon and sardines with bones), tea, small amounts in animal foods

RDA
1.5 to 4 mg (estimated)

ALLIES
Vitamin C and D, calcium, magnesium, phosphorus, fat

ANTAGONISTS
Salt, aluminum, vitamin C deficiency, sweating

DEFICIENCIES CAN CAUSE
Teeth and bone problems

NEED INCREASED WITH
Osteoporosis and osteoarthritis; periodontal disease, although no safe method has been developed which avoids toxicity

IODINE

FUNCTION
Necessary for proper function of thyroid (which regulates rate of oxidation within cell) and metabolism of all nutrients;

40 Nutrition in Nursing: The New Approach

essential for proper growth, energy, and metabolism; converts carotene to vitamin A

SOURCES
Seaweed and other plants grown near the sea; seafood, iodized salt, sea salt, mushrooms, fish-liver oil, drugs, food additives

RDA
Adults: 150 mcg

ALLIES
Calcium, magnesium, phosphorus, vitamin D

ANTAGONISTS
PCBs and lithium

DEFICIENCIES CAN CAUSE
Goiter, apathy, sensitivity to cold, enlargement of thyroid, weight gain, thickening of skin, hair loss, mental retardation, thyroid cancer

NEED INCREASED WITH
People in iodine-deficient areas, puberty, lactation and pregnancy, those on lithium

MOLYBDENUM

FUNCTION
Essential to function of enzymes involved in production of uric acid and oxidation of liver xanthine, aldehydes and sulfites; promotes growth; mobilizes release of iron from liver stores; helps prevent cavities

SOURCES
Yogurt, acidophilus, legumes, organ meats, grains, dark leafy greens

RDA
Required in trace amounts

ALLIES
Iron

ANTAGONISTS
Sulfur, copper, tungsten, refined grains

DEFICIENCIES CAN CAUSE
Decreased liver and intestinal xanthine oxidase activities; neurological abnormalities; displaced ocular lenses; lethal defect in sulfur metabolism; esophageal cancer; sexual impotency in older males

NEED INCREASED WITH
Those who have anemia, poor dentition (if excess cavities), gouty arthritis

VANADIUM

FUNCTION
Linked with lithium metabolism and enzymes; may reduce excess sodium levels; works with zinc in cell reproduction; depresses manufacture of cholesterol; helps prevent tooth decay; influences lipid metabolism, can substitute for molybdenum in certain processes

SOURCES
Fish, fats, vegetable oils, water, grains

RDA
Not established, but estimated to be 0.1 to 0.3 mg

ALLIES
Not established

ANTAGONISTS
Food processing

DEFICIENCIES CAN CAUSE
Slow healing, hair loss, premature aging

NEED INCREASED WITH
Aging; for those with high cholesterol; essential for those on purified diets—may be important in space travel

NICKEL

FUNCTION
Biological relevance uncertain, but may activate liver enzymes; may involve hormone, fat and membrane metabolism; may contribute to stabilization of nucleic acids

SOURCES
Seafood, cereals, grains, beans, vegetables

RDA
Not established, but estimated to be 0.3 to 0.6 mg

ALLIES
Vitamin B6, copper, zinc

ANTAGONISTS
High protein

DEFICIENCIES CAN CAUSE
Impaired iron absorption; retarded growth; reduction of blood hemoglobin; reduced blood glucose; decreased fertility; increased liver lipids

NEED INCREASED WITH
Heavy sweating, cirrhosis of liver; physiological stress; chronic kidney failure; essential for those on purified diets—may be important in space travel

ARSENIC

FUNCTION
Biological relevance uncertain; takes part in some reactions involving phosphate

SOURCES
Ubiquitous—found in high amounts in additives and weed killers

RDA
Not established, because of individual differences in susceptibility, but 43 micromolecules a day accepted as upper limit of safety

ALLIES
Low vitamin C levels; processed-food diet

ANTAGONISTS
Vitamin C; detoxifying foods such as complex carbohydrates

DEFICIENCIES CAN CAUSE
Low growth rate, pathologic changes in various organs

Trace amounts necessary, but the reason not understood

Bibliography

Ballentine, R. *Diet and Nutrition: A Holistic Approach* (Honesdale, Pa.: The Himalayan International Institute, 1978).

Bogert, L. J.; Briggs, G. M.; and Calloway, D. H. *Nutrition and Physical Fitness*, 8th ed. (Philadelphia: W. B. Saunders Co., 1960).

Burton, B. T. *Human Nutrition: A Textbook of Nutrition in Health and Disease* (New York: McGraw-Hill Book Company, 1976).

Fennema, O. "Principles of Food Science, part 1." In: *Food Chemistry*. (New York: Marcel Dekker, 1976).

Nutritonal Biochemistry and Pathology, vol. 3 (New York: Plenum Press, 1980).

Williams, R. J. *Physicians' Handbook of Nutritional Science* (Springfield, Ill.: Charles C. Thomas, 1978).

Wurtman, R. J. and Wurtman, J. J. *Nutrition and the Brain: Toxic Effects of Food Constituents on the Brain*, vol. 4 (New York: Raven Press, 1979).

2

PATIENT ASSESSMENT

The stress experienced ... today must be different from that experienced in the past, and the stress experienced by a member of a developed industrial society different from that experienced by a member of a developing and predominantly rural society.

TOM COX, M.D.

Nutrition courses taught in medical and nursing schools usually focus on an extreme disease process (for example, diabetes), or a surgical problem (for example, colostomy). Rarely, if ever, is a physician or nurse taught the nuances of subclinical nutrient deficiencies. Rarely, if ever, does a doctor or nurse learn how nutrition relates to *healing*.

Who should be responsible for the nutritional and emotional care of patients? If the food service group is in charge of nutritional care, that group must be patient-oriented rather than catering-oriented. However, in contrast to other hospital departments with direct impact on patient care, food services often has no direct or continuing accountability for its professional activities. So, until food service groups begin providing better nutritional care, and the horror of hospital malnourishment becomes a thing of the past, you as the primary caretaker can, and should, make certain that your patients are receiving good nutritional care. The important question to ask is: How can the nurse determine the patient's nutritional needs? (It is important to remember that stress and emotions deplete nutrients; therefore, they must be taken into account when treating any patient.)

Identifying nutritional needs

Although in recent years attitudes toward the nutritional support of hospitalized patients have changed for the better, the changes have not been remarkable, nor have they been widely practiced. The patient's hospital stay still involves mostly diagnostic procedures and physical care. Rarely does the physician take responsibility for nutritional treatment, especially if the patient doesn't have clear symptoms of malnutrition. The provision of nutritional support is a complex, multidisciplinary and multidepartmental activity. In the absence of such provision, the nurse must be well informed and creative.

The very idea that patients are not being supplied with basic nutritional needs is deplorable. Dr. Bjorn Isaksson of the department of clinical nutrition in Sahlgren's Hospital, Sweden, says, "It must be regarded as unacceptable that the most natural form of nutrition care—the general hospital diet—may cause malnutrition among patients who are forced to be hospitalized for more than one to two weeks, and, before proper nutrition support is given, signs of malnutrition must be evident." Studies in the United States show that malnutrition is widespread among patients hospitalized longer than two weeks. In some cases, treatment itself is associated with specific patterns of nutritional imbalance. *Much of it is avoidable.*

The lifesaving virtues of nutritional support and rehabilitation are more than anecdotal. Yet despite the rich storehouse of knowledge, the hospital continues to be one of the worst places for the consumption of health-promoting foods. If the patient was not malnourished on entering the hospital, malnourishment is almost always a consequence of the hospital stay. In fact, *the longer a patient is hospitalized, the more severe the malnourishment.* Studies conducted in Scandinavian hospitals in the 1970s indicate that the average patient is at risk to develop malnutrition during hospitalization. At the Twelfth International Congress of Nutrition, Dr. George L. Blackburn stated that "greater detection and prevention-reversal of malnutrition would go far in reducing morbidity, especially infectious and respiratory complications and wound dehiscence, resulting in shorter hospital stays and reduced need for respiratory therapy, intensive care units, and antibiotics."

Malnutrition in hospitals is not confined to degenerative diseases such as cancer, but is common to a broad category of diseases. It is very important to detect patients at nutritional risk. And when you do detect nutritional problems, it is often difficult to convince the patient, physician and dietician that there is a problem. For example, physicians often consider malnutrition in terms of symptoms rather than as a state of nourishment. They believe that if the patient has no symptoms of malnutrition, he or she does not need nutrients! And intertwined with this misunderstanding is an inability to detect the more subtle symptoms of nutritional deficiencies.

THE GREATEST NEED, THE LEAST AVAILABILITY

Of all the people in the world, the patient has the highest nutrient needs. Diseasae itself alters the way the body accepts and uses nutrients, and thus increases nutritional needs. Needs above normal are found in patients with impaired intestinal function, increased losses of nutrients from drug therapy, decreased anabolic processes and/or increased catabolic reactions. Such conditions are common after trauma or surgical intervention. Studies of patients in a metabolic ward show that most of them are not in nitrogen balance. We could cite example after example.

Hospitalized patients often have a poor appetite. It has been suggested that it is better to provide several small meals scattered over as large a part of the day as possible, thereby reducing the night's fast to less than ten to eleven hours. Patients with an impaired sense of smell (common among older people) find cold foods more palatable than hot foods. It is important to offer foods that are required for the healing process, but it is even more important that the patient eats that food.

Charts provide a record of temperature, blood pressure, medication use, and so on. Why not record how much or what kind of food a patient is consuming? Perhaps the doctor will notice and ask questions, or, better yet, perceive correlations, and eventually regard nutritional support as an important medical tool. When a patient is not eating, you have an excellent opportunity to discuss nutrition with the doctor. (You are the one who will note the lack of appetite, not the physician.)

Unless there is a policy against it, you might suggest that visitors bring food to the patient for two reasons:

First, eating alone in bed is not conducive to a hearty appetite under the best of circumstances. We all know that eating is a social activity. Why not encourage eating during visiting hours?

Second, institutional food processing often depletes nutrients. Overcooking—food preparation at too high a temperature or for too long a time, is very common in institutional cooking. Food is often left standing at hot temperatures.— These factors affect many nutrients. In addition, comparative studies on food preparation and exposure to air have shown that there is a relationship between the decrease in ascorbic acid and the substances responsible for taste. Tasteless, unappetizing foods and impaired taste reactions. will always make it more difficult to combat hospital malnutrition.

RECOGNIZING DEFICIENCIES

Gross symptoms of undernutrition are often obvious (big, bloated belly despite skinny arms and legs, yellow skin, and so on). Detecting more subtle symptoms requires more knowledge. Too often our prejudices and personal habits govern our points of view. (You know the old joke: any patient that weighs ten pounds more than the doctor is overweight.)

If you have read the "Deficiency can cause . . ." sections of the Nutrient Charts, you will know more than most professionals about the etiology of nutritional deficiencies. The following list cites only those symptoms that are overt—apparent by looking at a patient. The symptom does not necessarily mean that the patient suffers from the deficiency noted, but the chances are high that he or she does.

Condition	Deficiency
SKIN	
Dry skin	Vitamin A, polyunsaturated fatty acids
Pigmentation	Niacin
Petechiae, purpura, corkscrew hairs	Ascorbic acid
Acne	Riboflavin, pyridoxine (B6), zinc
Seborrheic dermatitis at nose	Riboflavin
Dermatitis	Niacin, pyridoxine (B6)
Eczema	Pantothenic acid
Grayish skin color	Biotin
ORAL	
Inflamed tongue	Vitamin A and/or B-complex, folic acid
Glossitis	Niacin, riboflavin, B12, folate, iron
Swollen, bleeding gums	Ascorbic acid
Red tongue	Niacin
Lesions on lips	Riboflavin
Cracks in corner of mouth	Riboflavin
Bad breath	Niacin, zinc
Canker sores	Niacin
Cheilosis (dry scaling of lips and angles of mouth)	B6, niacin, riboflavin
HAIR, NAILS	
Hair easily pluckable, sparse, dull	Protein
Spoon-shaped nails	Iron
White spots on nails	Zinc
Hair loss	Pantothenic acid, folic acid, biotin, inositol, iodine, vanadium

Condition	Deficiency
EYES	
Dull, dry conjunctiva	Vitamin A
Blepharitis (inflammation of eyelids)	B-complex
Ophthalmoplegia (paralysis of eye muscles)	Thiamin
Conjunctivitis	Biotin
Eye styes	Vitamin A
MISCELLANEOUS	
Bruises	Vitamin C
Edema	Vitamin C, pyridoxine (B6)
Muscle twitch	Magnesium
Delayed healing and tissue repair	Vitamin C, zinc, protein

Vitamin deficiencies are prominent in this list of visible symptoms. To the best of current knowledge, minerals play a greater role in systemic problems—those involving blood, cardiac, skeletal, gastrointestinal, sensory, glandular, fertility, sugar metabolism and central nervous system disorders. The range of trace elements and their importance has been discovered only in the last two decades. Perhaps future studies will find interrelationships between vitamins and minerals.

Symptoms of overt nutritional deficiency may be much more extensive than those listed above. In addition, precise information on the frequency and severity of nutritional imbalances is often difficult to come by because of wide differences in the duration of illness and varied aspects of treatment. So although assessing nutritional deficiency isn't an easy task, nutrition should still be at the heart of health care. Furthermore, the patient must become an informed partner and participant in the healing process. He or she should not be reduced to an object being repaired.

As a nurse, you may be asking yourself whether you should be imparting information of this sort. Many nurses are reluctant to intervene in lifestyle patterns; they question whether patients are ready to embrace major changes in a hospital setting. On the contrary, we believe this is the *best* time to impart nutritional counseling. A diet change may help resolve the health crisis. Education is the beginning. Help your patients learn.

Basic causes of malnutrition

The body is, in the most literal sense, the product of its nutrition. How many times have you heard, "But I eat balanced meals. I don't smoke or drink, I play tennis, and I even eat vegetables and take vitamins. Why have I become sick?" The answer lies in part in our failing foodways system. Although inheritance plays a role, we believe that genetic weaknesses may be intercepted with proper nourishment. Here is a brief overview describing various ways in which we are nutritionally shortchanged:

1 Soil may be contaminated with poisons, or depleted of necessary nutrients. For example, food grown close to busy highways contain high levels of lead; soil that is chemically fertilized is often selenium-deficient.

2 Improper food storage causes potato carcinogens, wheat and peanut fungus and bacterial growth.

3 Contaminated foods are rampant—swordfish with mer-

Patient Assessment 53

cury; seed grain with organic mercury; pigs with methyl mercury; rice with cadmium; wheat with selenium; oils with antiknock; milk with bacteria; apples with the carcinogenic hormone *alar*.

4 Food processing is responsible for significant nutrient losses. The milling of grain removes or reduces vitamins and minerals; technical errors are frequently made; freezing (with chelators) reduces trace elements in commercial green vegetables; sterilization of foods in jars and cans removes vitamin C and pyridoxine; canning may add tin, lead, and cadmium to foods; aluminum added to food in cooking causes contamination (especially when the food is acidic, like tomatoes).

5 Water used in rehydrating foods or in soft drinks may be contaminated with excess copper, cadmium or lead. Bacteria, fluoride and chlorine present problems, as do nitrates from surface drainage.

Specific causes of malnutrition are diarrhea, nausea, operations, parasites, food allergy, prematurity, vitamin dependence, chronic infection, pregnancy and lactation (unless the diet is superior), malabsorption, crash diets, bad eating habits, medications, biochemical individual differences or *any disease state*.

In addition to these factors, undesirable practices in the hospital affect nutrition, both directly and indirectly. These are:

1 failure to record height and weight;

2 rotation of staff at frequent intervals;

3 prolonged use of glucose and saline intravenous feedings;

4 withholding meals because of diagnostic tests;

5 ignorance of the composition of vitamin mixtures and other nutritional products;

6 unwarranted reliance on antibiotics for recovery from infection; and

7 limited availability of laboratory tests to assess nutritional status; failure to use those that are available.

The delay of nutrition support until the patient is in an advanced state of depletion can lead to irreversible problems. Patients who are malnourished tend to have delayed wound healing and greater susceptibility to infection and other complications.

Again, *it doesn't have to be this way!*

Identifying emotional needs

If given a choice, most people would certainly prefer going to the hospital for treatment to serving actively in war. But those same people might prefer appearing before the IRS to going to the hospital. The point is that going to the hospital is often compared with some of life's most threatening and upsetting experiences.

Patients don't know what to expect when they enter the hospital. They often feel depersonalized and dehumanized. Professionals on the hospital staff may have minimal time to calm fears, answer questions or allow for a patient's preferences. As dignity disappears, suspicion, fear and anxiety take its place.

As you well know, the nurse can have an enormous impact on the patient's morale and health. You may not have all the answers (even if the patient has the courage to ask the questions), but your insight and thoroughness can be of great benefit.

STRESS AND THE PATIENT

Stress is not always obvious from appearance or behavior. It would be easier if the patient wore a big sign that read, "I am scared to death." You really don't have to ask a patient if he or she is nervous. You can take it for granted that, at the very least, "ill-at-ease" gets packed with the suitcase.

Stress is not so much what is happening, but how one responds to what is happening—what is anticipated for tomorrow in addition to what actually happened yesterday. Although the physiological pathways involved in stress and physical breakdown are explored in detail later on, the point should be made now that stress affects wellbeing because it reduces the body's store of nutrients.

You may note these signs of stress in your patients:

Subjective effects. Anxiety, apathy, depression, fatigue, frustration, moodiness, nervousness, insomnia, pain.

Behavioral effects. Emotional outbursts, accident proneness, loss of appetite, excitability, impaired speech, nervous laughter, restlessness, trembling.

Cognitive effects. Frequent forgetfulness, hypersensitivity, mental blocks.

Physiological effects. Increased blood glucose levels, increased heart rate and blood pressure, dryness of mouth, sweating, dilation of pupils, difficulty breathing, hot and cold spells, "a lump in the throat," numbness and tingling in parts of the limbs.

Health effects. Chest and back pains, diarrhea, faintness and dizziness, frequent urination, headaches, nightmares, insomnia, skin rash.

You have the power to change the patients perception by changing the level of awareness of the hospital environment; and by teaching coping exercises. Obviously you don't have time for extensive psychotherapy or relaxation training sessions with each patient. But the ability to cope with stress can increase by applying a number of relaxation techniques.

One such technique involves the use of imagery. Dr. Charles Stroebel, in his book *QR: The Quieting Reflex*, describes a six-second technique for coping with stress anytime, anywhere. Although the mastery of the method may take a while, its application matches the speed of computer responses. Part of the training program involves conjuring up this image:

> Imagine that you are climbing aboard your own very safe spaceship. Feel your body sitting down in the control chair. After getting comfortable, imagine the objects in your spaceship. You are taking off. You are beginning to feel the increasing gravity. You feel the pressure against you. Your body is tense. Grip the arms of your chair to brace against the force of gravity. Inhale a deep breath. Hold it. Your whole body is getting more and more tense. Tighten your toes, feet, and legs. Tighten your fingers, arms, and shoulders. Tighten your neck and face. Hold on! You are tight and tense; the gravity is increasing; the tension is growing harder and tighter. Now as you suddenly burst through the gravity field, exhale deeply. You're weightless. Your whole body loosens. Let your jaw, tongue, and shoulders go loose. Let your eyes smile. Let your neck and shoulders go loose. Your arms and fingers go limp. Your abdomen, thighs, and legs go loose. Your ankles, feet, and toes are heavy and loose and warm. Feel your muscles letting go as you float. Your body is weightless and safe. You feel serene. Say to yourself, "Alert mind, effortless body." Notice how you feel when your muscles let go, when you feel

calm and serene. Your body has now floated safely back to where you began. You feel heavy, safe, and calm. Your body is sinking deeper and deeper into your chair. You feel heavy and calm. Stay completely motionless. Without actually doing it, think about lifting up one leg. Think about the muscles that you would have to use if you were to raise your arm. Notice the tensions that have crept into these muscles just because of your thoughts. Thoughts can invade your muscles to make you feel tense or to make you feel calm.

Using this example as a model, you can develop your own ideas. Anyone can learn relaxation, and it is an effective way to release stress. If aches and pains have been caused by extreme muscle tension, they can be prevented or alleviated with relaxation techniques. The threshold of pain tolerance can be raised. Relaxation can induce feelings of calm.

Here are several quick-acting techniques, which are "one-minute" vacations:

- Take three deep, slow breaths in through the nose and exhale slowly through pursed lips. Be aware of the life in the oxygen you are bringing in.
- Imagine you are falling through the chair or bed. Your entire being loosens.
- Imagine your body is resting on the bed and every inch is gently supported by the bed.
- Imagine you are a rag doll with all the stuffing slowly oozing out.
- Pull your shoulders up to your head, and then let them drop. Next, breathe in deeply and slowly—let the air fill your abdomen and hold your chest quiet and motionless. Then exhale, slowly, through your nose.
- Remember an unforgettable moment on a beach. Warm winds brush past your cheeks. White fluffy clouds fill the sky.

Colorful sailboats glide over blue and purple waters in the distance. Soft rhythmical music diffuses the noise of conversation. You have a tropical fruit drink in your hand. You feel mellow and tranquil.

- Imagine you are a snowman—the kind you used to build on your front lawn when you were a kid. The sun is shining, and you are melting away. Butter. Putty. Yielding. That's you.
- Close your eyes and settle down. Breathe out, then in. Then exhale very slowly with a slight sigh, like a balloon slowly deflating. Repeat. Feel the tension begin to drain away as you breathe out.
- Imagine that you are looking at something in the distance. Then visualize something very close. Then let the scene focus on something in the middle.
- Curl up as tightly as you can. Next, stretch out as far as you are able, with your back arched and fingers stretched. Then relax.
- Shake your hands loosely as if you are flicking water from your fingers—first one hand, then the other, then both together.

Practice any or all of these exercises and begin to teach them to your patients—as you give a bath, administer an injection, mobilize them or perform other activities.

THE NOISE LEVEL

Did you know that noise can raise blood pressure? Noise is a common and potent source of discomfort. Many people who are in perfect health react negatively to loud noise, and when you are sick, a whisper can sound like a shout. Noise also becomes a significant stress factor for people who are already anxious. Those "Hospital: Quiet, Please" signs have been placed in the streets for good reason. The problem is that hospitals are noisy places without outside help.

While construction was going on in one particular hospital, patients who were subjected to construction noise remained in the hospital longer than those who were in quiet areas, despite similar illnesses. It is uncertain whether noise has a detrimental effect on healing or on the efficiency of the hospital staff. No doubt each of these factors plays a role.

There are two things you can do to help your patients. Try to limit noisy conversations with your colleagues, and recommend that your patients' families bring a radio and/or tape recorder to the hospital. Soft music (perhaps heard through a headset) is especially soothing and healing.

HELPING THE INSOMNIAC

Touch or massage is an effective way of helping the patient who cannot sleep. Most patients can lie face down or on one side to prevent tension from an arched back.

Begin with long strokes moving from the waist upwards towards the neck and shoulders. Move along the sides of the spine first and then fan outwards towards the shoulders. You can add some gentle kneading motions. Massage should be firm, because you want the patient to feel what you are doing.

Now you can use soothing, gentle strokes moving down from the neck and shoulders to the waist. Alternate hands, but always have one hand in contact with the patient's skin. This movement is lingering. Your strokes should become lighter and slower. Even if your patient doesn't fall asleep, you have promoted a feeling of relaxation.

Bibliography

Blackburn, G. L. "Prognostic Strength of Nutritional Assessment." In *Nutrition, Health and Disease and International Development: Symposia from the XII International Congress of Nutrition*, eds. A. E. Harper and G. K. Davis (New York: Alan R. Liss, 1981).

Butterworth, C. E. "Hospital Malnutrition: Introductory Remarks." In *Nutrition, Health and Disease and International Development*.

Callaway, C. W. et al. "Guidelines for a Committee on Nutritional Care of the Hospital Medical Board." *American Journal of Clinical Nutrition* 42(1985):906.

Cox, T. *Stress* (Baltimore: University Park Press, 1978).

Isaksson, B. "How to Avoid Malnutrition During Hospitalization." In *Nutrition, Health and Disease and International Development*.

Illich, I. *Medical Nemesis: The Expropriation of Health* (New York: Random House, 1976).

Pfeiffer, Carl C. *Mental and Elemental Nutrients: A Physician's Guide to Nutrition and Health Care* (New Canaan, Conn.: Keats Publishing, Inc., 1975).

Stroebel, C. F. *QR: The Quieting Reflex* (New York: G. P. Putnam's Sons, 1982).

3

NUTRIENTS VERSUS CALORIES VERSUS ABSORPTION

We must acknowledge that our country has made very many mistakes in departing from natural nutrition. We must mend our ways for the evolution of the total acceptance of improved eating for today's healing and tomorrow's new generations.
SERAFINA CORSELLO, M.D.

Patients who are burn victims, have cancer or who have diabetes all have different nutritional needs, yet are given food with more attention to calorie counts than nutrition. Nutrients are not directly related to calories; thus, calorie counting is irrelevant. This chapter discusses why calories are a poor indicator of nutrient density. It also outlines the conditions necessary for the absorption of nutrients.

The Royal Infirmary in Bristol, England studied the effects of ingesting apples as compared with applesauce and apple juice. The results showed that an apple is ingested more than *ten times faster* in the form of extracted apple juice than when it is contained within the fibrous architecture of the whole apple. In the form of applesauce, it is ingested nearly *three times faster*. These findings confirm that the natural fiber of the whole apple slows the ingestion of nutrients. Since no chewing is required in the consumption of applesauce, the process is speeded up.

The study showed that apples are more satisfying than applesauce, which in turn is more satisfying than juice. The increased satiety from the apples and the applesauce lasted at least two hours. These data indicate that the satisfying effect of an apple is due as much to its fiber content as to its carbohydrate content, suggesting that extra satiety is partly dependent on the need to chew fiber. What is surprising is that the body handles the apple differently not only when the fiber is removed (as in the apple juice), but also when the fiber has been merely physically disrupted (as in the applesauce).

There are other disturbances too. When ingesting applesauce and apple juice, there is a higher level of insulin in the blood and a corresponding drop in blood sugar levels that does not occur after consuming the "natural" meal of a whole apple. So, the removal or disruption of fiber from a natural food can result in faster and easier ingestion, decreased satiety and disturbed glucose balance. Digesting refined carbohydrates, in the form of sugar or juice, requires more metabolic activity (including nutrient utilization of vitamins and minerals) than digesting complex carbohydrates, as the whole fruit.

You can see how calories are an overrated aspect of the diet. Perhaps calorie counting became popular because calories are more quantifiable and understandable than the intricacies of nutrient absorption, even if they are irrelevant compared to nutrients.

Immunity tips the balance between a disease-free state and a disease process. *Nutritional deficiency is the most common cause of secondary impairment of immunocompetence.* Despite this fact, sick people, healing people, pre-op and post-op patients are rarely given the nourishment they require.

Because of our work with nurses (we present "New Age" healing and nutrition seminars), we were recently interviewed about nutrition awareness among nurses and doctors. The interviewer asked us if physicians were still working with the RDAs and the four food groups. We couldn't help but respond that such knowledge would almost be an improvement. Most health professionals (as well as the lay public) count calories, not nutrients (if anything is counted at all). Persons with diabetes are placed on diets with a certain number of calories. Low-fiber diets are ordered for anyone with gastrointestinal problems, and soft diets for many other conditions. Clear and full liquids are ordered for post-surgical diets, even though the patient winds up with highly refined sugar substances. Milk and meat are favorite protein sources. We all know humans require a range of nutrients—including high fiber and quality protein—to avoid malnutrition. But it seems that this knowledge is forgotten in the case of patients.

The following paradigm is not uncommon: a patient's food intake is well below a desirable level. Depending on the degree of underfeeding and the length of that state, symptoms of malnutrition may occur. Some form of alternative nutrition may then be prescribed by the doctor, such as formulas, milkshakes or tube feedings, all while counting calories. With any luck, the patient becomes rehabilitated, and the physician thinks he or she has given the patient excellent nutritional support. This may be true, but it happens too late.

It is time to clear the air! All recommendations for patients should be made in terms of nutrient density of the daily diet. This kind of diet should meet the most critical needs.

"Balanced" nutrition

Diet is the food you eat. Nutrition is the study of what happens to food after you eat it; what the food does for you or what it does to you. According to Webster, nourishment is "that which sustains with substances necessary to life and growth." Optimal nourishment is that which sustains with substances necessary to life and growth in a most exemplary way. If you put regular gas in a car designed to run on high-test fuel, the car will run, but you'll know the difference. In much the same way, humans function better on optimal nourishment.

A manufacturer advertises that its frozen yogurt bar has more "balanced nutrition" than an eight-ounce portion of yogurt. Since fat and sugar are the main ingredients in the bar (yogurt places fifth), you may wonder how the company can make this claim. The claim is based on an assumed definition of "balanced nutrition." The manufacturer maintains that balanced nutrition means a lot of vitamins and minerals, and disregards other substances in the product.

Another company advertises that its variety of potato chips has calories equivalent to those in a cup of milk, and has the same amount of salt as in two slices of bread. These statements are true. But do the chips contribute to balanced nutrition?

Commercial peanut butter contains partially hydrogenated fat. When unsaturated fat is hydrogenated, it may be as harmful as the saturated fats. Large quantities of unsaturated fats are also harmful. Many commercial peanut butters are heavily endowed with sugar. Some have molasses in addition to sugar, plus chemical emulsifiers to prevent the oil from separating and to extend the shelf life of the product. The germ or heart of the peanut is often removed in processing. (The germ is the little bump you see when you separate the two parts of the nut. The germ spoils quickly, but it is the part that has very high nutrient value.) Nine percent of the fat in peanut butter is saturated, despite advertising which gives you an entirely different impression. Balanced nutrition?

Twenty-two percent of the fat in margarine is saturated. Margarine has the same amount of fat as butter. But margarine contains an unnatural, distorted fat. Margarine also has artificial butter-like flavor, odor and color, as well as chemical protectors and preservatives. (Compare the label of margarine with non-dyed butter, and you decide which you want to eat.) Balanced nutrition?

Advertising has convinced everyone that it is unAmerican to start the day without a glass of orange juice—regardless of where you live. The people of Montana have been convinced that they must have oranges, even though they live long distances from orange groves. If fruits and vegetables are going to travel, they must be picked before they are ripe. This prevents them from spoiling on their pilgrimage to faraway states. However, when a fruit or vegetable is picked before it is fully ripe, it does not have its full complement of nutrients. Green oranges are often dyed orange, and many oranges are coated with mineral oil or carnauba wax. Balanced nutrition?

Wheat flour is especially ravaged by processing. In the refining process, more than half of each of the most essential nutrients are deleted. The milling process destroys 40 percent of the chromium present in the whole grain, as well as 86 percent of the copper, 78 percent of the zinc and 48 percent of the molybdenum. By the time the flour is completely refined, it has lost most of its phosphorus, iron and thiamine, and a good deal of its niacin and riboflavin. And its crude fiber content has been cut down considerably.

White flour has been plundered of most of its vitamin E, important oils and protein amino acids. After the wheat is stripped of its nutrients, the flour is bleached, the shortening is altered with sweetening agents (dextrose, refined sugar and corn syrup), the dough is stretched further with chemicals and synthetic yeast nutrients are added. The bread usually has a freshener added to it. Balanced nutrition?

Children and dieticians are still being taught that eating foods from the four food groups provides balanced nutrition. Before we tampered with food, the four-food-group diet worked. The four-food-group approach to nutrition is outdated and misleading. A "balanced diet" is the presumed result of choosing from four arbitrarily defined groups of food. Note these possible selections of foods from the four food groups:

Meat group. Fast-food frankfurter; breakfast sausages; fast-food hamburger; cold cuts; sausages; feedlot steaks.

Vegetable group. Canned or frozen vegetables; prepackaged mashed potatoes; French fries; potato chips; sauerkraut.

Dairy group. Ice cream; milk shakes; whipped cream; processed cheese; milk that has been heated under high temperatures (pasteurization) and has gone through a process that disturbs the molecular structure of the fat particles (homogenization).

Grain group. White bread; pancakes; muffins; corn chips; packaged dry and sweetened cereals; cakes and cookies; white rice.

One more group is ignored—a group now referred to as "other," which includes hydrogenated fats, refined sugar, excessive salts, nitrates and artificial colors and flavors. The trouble is that this other group pervades the first four groups. Just because the food industry tells us that it's okay to consume these foreign molecules doesn't mean that it is okay. Balanced nutrition?

Nutrients are lost when foods are gassed, waxed, dyed, soaked, peeled and/or overcooked—processes used when food is frozen, canned, and bottled, and then stored and recooked. Canned or frozen food no longer contains its original nutrient content. If food sits around for several months without benefit of these processing steps, it would not look, smell or taste like food fit for human consumption.

Perhaps you, like most Americans, have been duped by Madison Avenue advertising and believe that vegetables to be frozen are picked at the peak of ripeness and quickly flash-frozen. The fact is that vegetables are not routinely frozen immediately after harvest. Availability of processing doesn't always coincide with readiness to harvest, and delays in processing result in substantial losses of nutrients.

A study conducted by the Department of Agriculture demonstrated that the average frozen food changes temperature seventeen times. With each temperature change, there are additional nutrient losses. But that's the least of it.

Some form of blanching is usually essential to inactivate enzyme systems when products are prepared for freezing. Blanching may be carried out in either hot water or steam. Chemical or mechanical trimming and peeling procedures are also nutrient thieves. One of the most common techniques is that of lye-peeling where vegetables are treated with 1 percent alkali at about 200°F. Vegetables with loosened skins are then conveyed under high velocity jets of water which wash away lye and any residual skin.

Substantial amounts of the more labile nutrients are usually lost in the freezing process. These include vitamin C and thiamin (B1), both of which

1 cannot be stored in the body;
2 are subject to leaching during processing;
3 are highly susceptible to chemical degradation; and
4 are present in many foods but are often deficient in the diet.

Fifty percent of vitamin C and up to 60 percent of vitamin B1 can be lost in the freezing process. Specifically, water blanching causes a 30 percent loss of niacin from lima beans, a 50 percent loss of vitamin C from spinach, a 19 percent loss of riboflavin from green peas and a 14 percent loss of riboflavin from green beans.

Storage, as already indicated, continues to take its toll on nutrients. Such losses vary with the product and increase with time. Both fresh and frozen vegetables lose nutrients when cooked, but the time of frozen storage prior to cooking may cause additional cooking losses.

And if you did get food that was not mushed, mashed and mangled, chances are your patients (and you, like most

Americans) derive more than 30 percent of your calories from nutritionally poor sources such as soft drinks and snack foods—which create malnutrition by displacing more nourishing foods in the diet. The calorie count goes on oblivious to these alterations in nutrients.

Nutrient-dense foods

Nutrient-dense foods are foods which are high in vitamins and minerals, contain oils in their natural form and can boast high-quality protein. The avocado is an example of a nutrient-dense food, high in essential fatty acids, vitamin E and many other important nutrients, but it is better known for its "high" calorie content and summarily relegated to a low-priority position. The more nutrient-dense foods in a patient's diet, the easier the healing process. The master key is a *variety* of nutrient-dense foods. Excessively high protein diets are hazardous to individuals who are not exercising or who do not have large bodies. RDAs do not allow for immobility or compromised digestive systems.

Here are a few factors which affect the nutrient value of food:

- Iron absorption can be inhibited by large intakes of chocolate, cola and other caffeine-containing beverages.

- A diet high in fat increases phosphorus absorption and lowers calcium levels.

- Excessive amounts of unsaturated fatty acids (oils found in Italian salad dressings, peanut oils, safflower oils, and so forth) can produce a deficiency in vitamin E.

- Vegetables grown in selenium-depleted soil may result in selenium deficiency, which is known to cause liver damage.
- Baking soda destroys thiamin (vitamin B1).
- Antibiotics are antagonistic to many of the B vitamins.
- Diets too high in protein deplete calcium and vitamin B6 levels.
- Freezing foods affects pantothenic acid.
- Exposure to air and heat, storage and processing destroys vitamin C.
- Storing food at room temperature is destructive to folic acid.
- The average American diet has a negative effect on chromium. (Remember, this is the only country with chromium deficiencies.)
- High quantities of bran destroy manganese.
- Minerals compete with each other. Excess zinc, calcium, cadmium, and iron affect copper levels.

You are *not* what you eat

Humans have always been intrigued by the mystery of what happens to food after it is eaten. High technology is helping us solve that mystery. Although there are still many gaps and unanswered questions, there are a few basic easily understood steps. These are:

Ingestion. The actual taking of food into the body. Culture, economy, emotions, hunger and appetite all play a role in determining what and how much a person will eat. Studies show that people do not necessarily select what is good, but rather what is liked.

The mouth masticates food and begins the digestive process with ptyalin, an enzyme that acts on starches. The esophagus leads to the stomach and functions as a connective tube.

Digestion. The release of nutrients from food; a hydrolytic process. Insoluble foods are "broken down" into smaller particles by the addition of water. The stomach holds food until the digestive process continues. The small intestine is subdivided into three areas—the duodenum, the jejunum and the ileum—and is the longest part of the digestive tract. The final stages of digestion take place in the small intestine.

Absorption. The end products of digestion; also, the passage of food through the gastrointestinal tract through the villi of the small intestine. After absorption, nutrients are circulated either by blood alone, or in the case of fats, by the lymph and then the blood.

Utilization. Transportation of nutrients by the blood to all cells of the body. The nutrients serve the body in various ways as needed. This process, although orderly, is highly complex. Utilization is facilitated by additional changes or reactions with other substances. These may take place at many sites, including the individual cell, the liver or the kidney. Some nutrients are stored for future use, and others are excreted.

Many factors exert a marked influence on food from the time it is ingested until it is utilized.

Foods are not usually absorbed through the digestive tract before they are broken down into small molecules. Small quantities, however, are absorbed as large molecules. This means that the body may treat foods as foreign bodies that can act immunologically when ingested as antigens, often causing antigen-antibody reactions. Thus, foods not only provide nutrition, but can also promote adverse effects. *The same food that nourishes can impair the immune system.* The adage "You are what you eat" should be revised to *You are what you assimilate.*

A recent study of people who suffer from wheat sensitivity (and their numbers grow increasingly higher), has found that wheat protein contains a dietary antigen that can activate T-suppressor cell activity and impair the body's immune system. Incomplete breakdown products from reactive foods such as gluten from wheat or casein from milk are examples of foods that can be transported through the "leaky" gastrointestinal mucosa into systemic circulation. When these incomplete protein breakdown products are delivered to the bloodstream, they can be trapped in the liver or in joint spaces. This can initiate inflammatory processes that cause pain and edema. The physician rarely attributes these symptoms to food sensitivity. "Aging," on the other hand, is a common diagnosis. Even more serious is the fact that incomplete breakdown products do not deliver nutrients to the body, but add "empty" calories. So a glass of milk and a slice of toast, which contain calories, may in fact have a deleterious effect.

Foods that help the gastrointestinal mucosa work at peak efficiency and thus aid in the digestion and assimilation of nutrients are substances that reduce the relative load of dietary antigens. Vegetables, such as leafy greens, are examples of these foods. Improved digestion and assimilation would facilitate an improved immunological status.

We can help strengthen the immune system and promote tissue repair through the complex synergistic interaction of vitamins, minerals, amino acids and other constituent molecules without interference when we feed patients *nutrient-dense, hypoallergenic* foods.

The simple addition of acidophilus culture may improve nutrient absorption. Individuals who have suffered from indigestion, irritable bowel syndrome, colitis and excess acid stomach have found symptomatic relief from this cultured milk product. Acidophilus has a tonic effect on the intestinal tract, and because it does not promote diarrhea, it is not a true laxative. In addition, its bacteriostatic effect improves gastrointestinal function, favorably altering the pH of the bowel. Its beneficial effect might also be attributed to a reduction in the delivery of antigens to the gut mucosa.

Optimal diet

No one knows precisely what constitutes the optimal diet. Dr. Mark Hegsted, renowned nutritionist, says:

> The fact that we do not know the optimal solution cannot and does not prevent us from using whatever relevant evidence is available to make the best judgment possible. If we wait until we know everything we need to know, we will wait forever. The issue is not the definition of an optimal diet—the issue is whether or not current dietary practice can be improved.... The time to start is now.

Our idea of the optimal institutional diet is discussed with an awareness of what is available and desired.

The caring relationship

Nurses have a humanistic, altruistic concern for reducing human suffering and improving the quality of life; this attitude may even influence life expectancy. These goals can be achieved with an improved health care delivery system. Talking to the patient once is not sufficient. On the other hand, too many interactions between the patient and health-care professional are equally ineffective. (Research studies demonstrate that patient compliance is better in private practice than in the hospital or clinic because of a better-established relationship.) The nurse is in a unique position to work on that relationship.

We hope that the dietician will assume responsibility for the quality of nutritional care. The nurse should be allowed to educate the patient if he or she would like to do so. Needless to say, communication and cooperation among the entire hospital staff is essential for the hospitalized patient's wellbeing.

Before you can educate the patient about good nutrition, you must believe that education will make a difference. We advocate that each nurse personally follow an optimal diet for three weeks, even if the nurse self-starts the process. When you see what it does for someone in good health, you will be convinced that the benefits for hospitalized patients can be phenomenal.

Just think of what you can accomplish if you believe that all people can change, and you are able to convince your patients of this. To accomplish this goal you must be sensitive to the patient's feelings and experiences. To be completely successful, you will have to teach your patients how to be self-sufficient in following their diet. Remember that you are teaching a process, not a temporary solution. You have a few powerful assets: the patient is usually motivated by fear of long-term illness (or even death), he or she wants to get well and believes that the hospital experience will make him or her well.

The turn of the century marked an improvement in hospital sanitation even before it was known what specific microorganisms were associated with hospital infection. Although we need to know more about micro- and macronutrients, we do know that improved nutrition means faster healing and reduced risk of further disease. You must teach your patients the guidelines for good nutrition. By entering into a caring relationship with your patients, you can assist in modifying their food choices, and hasten the healing process. Who is in a better position to do this than you, the nurse?

Bibliography

Feinstein, A. *Journal of Chronic Diseases* 11(1960):349.

Fennema, O. "Effects of Freeze Preservation on Nutrients." In *Nutritional Evaluation of Food Processing,* eds. R. Harris and E. Karmas (Westport, Conn: AVI Publishing, 1977), pp. 244–288.

Haber, G. B.; Heaton, K. W.; and Murphy, D. "Depletion and Disruption of Dietary Fiber." *Lancet* 2(1977):679.

Hemmings, W. A. *Food Antigens and the Gut* (London: Lancaster Press, 1979).

O'Farrelly, C.; Whelan, C. A.; and Weip, D. "Suppressor-Cell Activity in Celiac Disease Induced by Alpha-Gliadin: A Dietary Antigen." *Lancet* 2(1984): 1305.

Stavney, L. S. et al. "Evaluation of the pH-Sensitive Telemetering Capsule in the Estimation of Gastric Secretory Capacity." *American Journal of Digestive Disorders* 10(1966):753.

4

NUTRIENT AND DRUG INTERACTIONS

I believe that nutritional side effects of drugs are preventable, and that most of them occur because physicians are unaware that they exist.

DAPHNE A. ROE, M.D.

We have established that malnutrition compromises the immune system. Drug-induced nutritional deficiencies are among the ten leading causes of malnutrition in the United States today. Although many nurses and physicians are aware that the side effects of some drugs may be worse than the symptoms they attempt to relieve, they do not always recognize that these side effects may contribute to nutritional deficiencies. The effects may be dose-related or dependent on the nutritional status of the patient.

How drugs affect nutrients

Drugs affect nutrients in several ways. They can:

1 impair the absorption of nutrients;
2 increase the excretion of nutrients;
3 decrease the utilization of nutrients; and
4 interfere with the transport of nutrients.

Indirectly, drugs may affect appetite and customary eating patterns. The route of administration, dosage schedule and satiation of the patient may also affect the distribution and metabolism of drugs. This in turn may change their pharmacological effects, and change their impact on nutrition as well.

When disease affects nutritional status the patient suffers even more. Almost all these patients are taking drugs, and almost all drugs cause nutrient losses. The patient suffers doubly.

Even substances applied topically can cause nutritional problems. A recent epidemic of skin poisoning in France affected several hundred children, thirty-six of whom died. The source of the toxic agent was talcum powder which, because of a manufacturing error, contained high levels of hexachlorophene. (Hexachlorophene has been banned in the United States. Frighteningly, old containers abound in many American bathroom cabinets.)

Phenytoin, an anticonvulsant found in Dilantin, can lower folate levels in many patients. This could have devastating effects and promote anemia. (Folate is a compound of the B vitamin complex.) But taking large amounts of folic acid to correct the deficiency may itself induce seizures. Elimination of seizures is the very reason the drug is administered in the first place. So you can see how complicated drug-nutrient effects can be. But few people, it seems, can avoid drug-induced nutritional problems. Even common aspirin can affect nutrition. Chronic use of salicylates has been shown both to decrease uptake of vitamin C in leukocytes and impair the protein-binding ability of folate.

Hoffmann La-Roche, Inc. uses full-page ads in leading medical journals to create an awareness of nutrient-drug interactions among physicians. The advertising statement defines the specific vitamin that is affected by a specific drug. The following are among the interactions listed:

Drug	*Vitamin Affected*	*Possible Manifestation and Mechanisms*
Mineral oil	A, D, K	Rickets
Cholestyramine (*to lower cholestrol such as Questran*)	Folacin, B12, A, D, K	Osteomalacia (bone and muscular weakness)
Colchicine (*for gouty arthritis*)	B12	Absorptive enzyme damage; damage to intestinal wall
Glutethimide (*Doriden, for temporary insomnia*)	D	Osteomalacia
Hydralazine (*Apresoline, for hypertension*)	B6	Peripheral nutropathy; increased excretion of vitamin/drug complex
Neomycin (*Mycifradin, for diarrhea*)	B12, A	Damage to intestinal wall; binding of bile salts; intrinsic factor inhibition
Penicillamine (*Cuprimine, for rheumatoid arthritis*)	B12	Peripheral neuropathy (nervous disorders of extremities)

Drug	Vitamin Affected	Possible Manifestation and Mechanisms
Potassium chloride (*Kayciel, to compensate for drug-induced deficiency*)	B12	Decreased ileal pH (condition of body fluids)
Salicylates (*aspirin*)	Folacin, C, K	Decreased protein binding; decreased uptake in thrombocytes and leukocytes
Sulphasalazine (*Azulfidine, for ulcerative colitis*)	Folacin	Decreased absorption
Tetracycline	C	Increased excretion

A recent article in the *New England Journal of Medicine* dramatically points out that medication which is used to treat one condition may cause an equally serious condition. All drugs have multiple actions; the principal action should be the benefit and the secondary action the side effects. But it doesn't always work that way. *There are no drugs without side effects. Only ineffective drugs can be completely safe.* Patients should be aware that taking any drug involves a delicate balance between risk and benefit. In addition, the number of side effects increase proportionally with the number of drugs the patient is consuming.

Nurses do not generally have the authority to order drugs, but they can monitor intended effects and side effects. When administering medication, nurses should be aware that they can advise patients of their right to refuse any drug that might be causing difficulties. (Needless to say, the physician should be notified.)

People have been searching for relief from pain and suffering for millennia, but the technological explosion of the last one hundred years has yielded many new medicines. Nurses in particular should understand the profound effect of medications on the patient's physical, mental and emotional states; the nurse should also be aware that patients have different drug-tolerance levels. It is the nurse's responsibility to note the effects that drugs have on the patient.

THE MUSHROOM PHENOMENON OF DRUGS

For the hospitalized patient, the necessary administration of medications is often a mushroom phenomenon. Unfortunately, most drugs are powerful chemical agents as alien to human tissues and metabolism as the noxious and toxic pollutants of our environment. The body recognizes most medicines as poisonous, and responds with biochemical mechanisms to neutralize and eliminate these foreign substances as rapidly as possible. This detoxification relies on enzymatic breakdown of the pharmaceutical compounds, whose presence increases the patient's dietary need for vitamin coenzymes. This elevated demand for nutrients increases the need for specific vitamins and can produce outright, or clinical, malnutrition if the diet fails to provide increased quantities of the necessary coenzymes. It is a dietary burden, or stress factor, that lasts as long as anyone continues to take a medication (for example, if the patient takes aspirin daily for the relief of arthritis pain and inflammation, the requirement for vitamin C is automatically increased as long as the analgesic is continued).

How can your knowledge of this information help the patient? You can encourage your patient to form a partnership with you; you can guide the patient until he or she learns self-care. At least 18 to 30 percent of all hospitalized patients end up with drug reactions that often double their stays in the hospital. Perhaps you can help change that statistic.

Be particularly aware that:

- Antibiotics (e.g. neomycin, tetracycline, penicillin and so forth) interfere with the absorption of fat-soluble vitamins (A and K) from the digestive tract into the circulatory system. Additional quantities of these vitamins may be necessary during drug therapy.

- Regular laxative use, particularly of mineral oil, interferes with the absorption of fat-soluble vitamins (A, D, E and K) from the digestive tract. Laxatives may result in loss of electrolytes, steatorrhea and decreased intestinal uptake of glucose. If a patient is taking mineral oil on a regular basis, be certain that he or she is receiving adequate quantities of these nutrients.

- Surfactants (e.g. dioctyl sodium sulfosuccinate, a fecal softener and Tween 80, an "inactive ingredient" in many liquid drug formulations) may increase absorption of cholesterol and vitamin A.

- Prolonged use of cholesterol-lowering drugs (e.g. Questran, cholestyramine, clofibrate) interferes with the absorption of fat-soluble vitamins A and D and water-soluble B12 from the gut. It also reduces the absorption of iron and sugar.

- Diabetics and people with hyperthyroid metabolism have difficulty converting beta-carotene (provitamin A from plant sources) into usable vitamin A. They may require supplementation with the preformed vitamin—particularly if they are being treated with insulin, oral hypoglycemics or thyroid medications.

Nutrient and Drug Interactions 83

- Anticonvulsant medications (e.g. Dilantin), phenobarbital, phosphate-containing laxatives and sleep-inducing drugs containing glutethimide (e.g. Doriden) increase the need for vitamin D if such drugs are taken on a regular basis, and make the patient prone to bone diseases.

- The mineral iron and various thyroid hormones are biochemical antagonists of vitamin E. Their regular use will increase the need for the nutrient. In contrast, E may enhance the blood-thinning effects of anticoagulants, such as Coumadin (more than therapeutically intended) and lead to internal hemorrhaging. Consult your physician about the simultaneous use of such drugs and vitamin E.

- Over-the-counter antacids tend to deplete the body's supply of water-soluble vitamins (C, B1, B2, B3, B6, B12, folic acid, biotin, cholines and pantothenic acid). Regular antacid use necessitates additional intake of these nutrients.

- Diuretics accelerate the flushing of water-soluble vitamins and minerals from the body. Frequent use of dehydrating drugs, such as diuretics, "water pills" and antihypertensives, raises the dietary requirement for vitamins C, B1, B2, B3, B12, folic acid and biotin. These nutrients may be an important nutritional adjunct to prolonged drug therapy.

- The frequent use of prescription analgesics (e.g. Indocin), or over-the-counter products (aspirin or other salicylate), anticoagulants (e.g. Coumadin), antidepressants (e.g. Permitil) and steroids (e.g. Cortisone), tends to increase the body's demand for vitamin C. Supplementation with the vitamin is probably advisable during therapy.

- Ascorbic acid (the usual form of vitamin C) makes urine more acidic, and in the presence of sulfa drugs (e.g. Gantrisin) may upset kidney chemistry. Use of ascorbate forms of the vitamin avoids this problem, but be certain to check with the patient and inform the physician of supplementation with C before any sulfa medication is started.

- Riboflavin (B2) and folic acid are important factors in the detoxification of methotrexate used in chemotherapy. Achieving a proper balance between these vitamins and the drug is critical to avoid nutritional deficiencies without reducing the therapeutic effectiveness of the medication.

- Daily use of antidepressants (e.g. Elavil), estrogens (e.g. Premarin), hydralazine-containing antihypertensives (e.g. Apresoline), isoniazid-containing drugs for the treatment of tuberculosis (e.g. Rifamate) and penicillamine-containing drugs for the treatment of arthritis all tend to increase the body's requirements for vitamin B6.

- Antigout medications containing colchicine (e.g. Colbenemid), anticoagulant drugs (e.g. Coumadin) and potassium supplements (e.g. Kaochlor, used to compensate for the loss of potassium during diuretic-antihypertensive drug therapy) tend to block absorption of vitamin B12 from the digestive tract. Colchicine may destroy or injure the intestinal epithelial lining. Supplementation with the vitamin may be wise.

- Chronic administration of glucocorticoids (cortisone-related drugs) may produce osteoporosis. People treated with large doses often develop more severe cases of the disease. The impaired skeletal growth and decreased bone mass may result in part from a block in intestinal absorption of calcium or a defect in vitamin D metabolism. Glucocorticoids also have been shown to decrease ascorbic acid levels in test animals. Whatever the mechanism, an excess decreases absorption of calcium and phosphorus, and at the same time increases their excretion.

- Estrogens in oral contraceptives interfere with polyglutamate conjugase, resulting in decreased absorption of dietary folic acid. Contraceptive pills in general decrease the physiologic levels of five other nutrients: riboflavin, pyridoxine, vitamin B12, ascorbic acid and zinc, and increase the levels of iron and copper.

- Antimicrobials (e.g. neomycin) bind fatty acids and bile acids and may cause steatorrhea. They may also decrease absorption of folic acid and vitamin B12.

- Irritating drugs (e.g. nitrofurantoin, phenylbutazone, aminosalicylic acid) may be administered with or immediately after meals to buffer the irritating effect. Other drugs (e.g. belladonna, propantheline and related anticholinergic agents) may be given shortly before a meal in an attempt to reduce gastric acid secretion and gut motility. Still others (e.g. antibiotics destroyed by gastric acidity such as penicillin G and erythromycin) are best administered at least one hour before or two hours after meals, so as to encounter the least acid environment and the shortest gastric emptying time.

- With certain drugs (e.g. sulfonamides), food delays, but does not decrease, gastrointestinal absorption. With others (e.g. penicillin G potassium), there is a definite decrease in both the rate and amount absorbed. With penicillin, food slows the rate of gastric emptying, permitting the drug to be exposed for a longer time to acid, which destroys the antibiotic. Tetracycline, on the other hand, is chelated by calcium found in foods (milk, cottage cheese), which interferes with absorption of the tetracycline. One study shows that warfarin absorption is inhibited by a substance found in cooking oil.

- Some drugs exhibit enhanced absorption (e.g. griseofulvin) when given with a high-fat meal. Some foods may cause acidification or alkalinization of the urine, thus altering the rate of excretion of certain drugs. These drugs may be given shortly before a meal in an attempt to reduce gastric acid secretion and gut motility.

• Nicotine can cause some drugs to break down chemically in the body more quickly. The Surgeon General reported in 1979 that "smoking of tobacco should be considered one of the primary sources of drug interactions." One such interaction involves caffeine. Caffeine in coffee is metabolized twice as fast by smokers as by nonsmokers.

In addition to these classified symptoms, many patients have idiosyncratic or hypersensitive reactions to drugs. Listen to your patients' complaints. Ask them to pay attention to unusual or different symptoms, and record these facts on the charts. This kind of attentive and caring attitude can go a long way toward finding the causes of problems and helping the patient get well.

Discuss coffee consumption with your patients. Caffeine plays a role in chronic fatigue and even heart disease. It affects the walls of blood vessels, blocks neuromodulators and can interfere with aspirin's antifever action.

Caution your patients not to use soda to wash down medications. Soft drinks destroy the effectiveness of antibiotics because of their acidity. The same is true for antihistamines and narcotic pain relievers like codeine.

Thalidomide produced a rare defect in high frequency and was easily recognized at birth. Yet it took 4000 to 5000 cases in Germany and from 1956 until 1961 to relate the effect to the drug. We mention this to demonstrate that less apparent damage done by other drugs goes unnoticed. Relationships are not always recognized quickly.

How nutrients affect drugs

Several foods can produce unexpected results for the patient on certain medications. A classic example is the effect of tyramine-containing foods on a patient taking monoamine oxidase inhibitors used to treat depression. Headache, nosebleeds, increased blood pressure and occasionally a cerebrovascular accident can result. Cheddar cheese and Gruyère cheese contain relatively large amounts of tyramine, as do most aged cheeses. Tyramine is also found in pickled herring and other aged protein foods.

Excessive amounts of green leafy vegetables rich in vitamin K may decrease the effectiveness of anticoagulants. Brussels sprouts and cabbage can cause clinical symptoms and an apparent interaction with thyroid-like drugs.

A possible source of excess sodium may be drinking water, either as a natural component of the water or as a substance added to soften "hard" water. Softening of Chicago water, which is moderately hard, adds about 120 mg sodium per liter.

Although food–drug interactions represent an area which is badly in need of research, you should be aware that such interactions do exist.

Drugs and the senior citizen

The elderly use hospitals at more than three times the rate of the rest of the American population. This group requires a great deal of assistance, particularly nursing care.

Many senior citizens take one or more medications on a daily basis, often for months or years at a time. It is thus important to know what additional demands are being made by the drugs so that dietary compensation, through foods or vitamin supplements, can be made. For example, any disease requiring extended bed rest causes rapid excretion of calcium.

It is difficult for an older person to shake off side effects and adverse reactions. Drug therapy that may not be very debilitating to a younger patient may "wipe out" an older patient.

Older people often require less sleep than usual, so what appears to be insomnia may be a normal pattern. Check this out with older patients who may be taking sleeping pills unnecessarily.

Decreased sensitivity to taste and smell often accompany old age, and some drugs will enhance the loss of taste acuity. Additional zinc often alleviates this problem.

See Chapter 5 for safe supplementation regimens.

Nutrient–nutrient interactions

Awareness of the effects of nutrient interactions is recent knowledge. Here are some examples:

- High-fiber diets may deplete minerals
- Vitamin C potentiates the absorption of iron
- Vitamin D is necessary for calcium utilization
- Magnesium and calcium "go" together
- Circulating levels of vitamin D respond to protein ingestion within one hour, and influence the excretion of calcium

This is the kind of helpful information you can impart to your patients where appropriate.

As reported by D. B. Clayson, two sets of test animals were exposed to a carcinogen. One set of animals had been fed a nutritionally *unbalanced* regimen. The first set became highly susceptible to cancer induced by the cancer-causing agent; the well-fed group had a much lower tumor incidence. Experiments like this support the general conclusion that the cells of a properly nourished individual are better able to detoxify harmful substances and to resist cancer.

The physician must be conscious of the need for supplemental nutrients when drug administration has increased the vitamin need beyond that which could be obtained through diet. There is a slowly advancing recognition that the provision of adequate nutrition is an essential adjuvant to all forms of treatment in the hospital. Is it too far-fetched to suggest that the nurse can educate the doctor?

Bibliography

Alfrey, A. "Aluminum Intoxication." *New England Journal of Medicine* 310(1984):1113.

Brin, M. "Drugs and Environmental Chemicals in Relation to Vitamin Needs." In *Nutrition and Drug Interrelations*, eds. T. N. Hathcock and J. Coon (New York: Academic Press, 1978).

Clayson, D. B. "Nutrition and Experimental Carcinogenesis: A Review." *Cancer Research* 35(1975):3292.

Favus, M. J. "Effects of Cortisone Administration on the Metabolism and Localization of 25-hydroxycholecalciferol in the Rat." *Journal of Clinical Investigation* 52(1973):1328.

Kamen, B. and Kamen, S. *Osteoporosis: What It Is, How to Stop It, How to Prevent It* (New York: Pinnacle, 1984; St. Martin's Press, 1986).

Hagerman, R. J. and Levitas, A. "Dilantin and the Fragile X Syndrome." *New England Journal of Medicine* 308(1983):1424.

Martin-Bouyer, G. "Outbreak of Accidental Hexachlorophene Poisoning in France." *Lancet* 1(1982):91.

Howe, J. C. et al. "The Postprandial Response of Vitamin D Metabolites in a Postmenopausal Woman." *American Journal of Clinical Nutrition* 39(1984):691.

Levy, S. J. *Managing the Drugs in Your Life* (New York: McGraw-Hill Book Co., 1983).

Melmon, K. L. "Preventable Drug Reactions: Causes and Cures." *New England Journal of Medicine* 284(1971):1361.

Ovesen, L. "Drugs and Vitamin Deficiency." *Drugs* 18(1979):278.

Raisz, L. G. and Kream, B. E. "Regulation of Bone Formation," part 2. *New England Journal of Medicine* 309(1983):83.

Roe, D. A. *Drug-Induced Nutritional Deficiencies* (Westport, Conn.: AVI, 1978), p. 26.

Vitale, J. J. "Nutrition and the Musculoskeletal System." In *Human Nutrition: A Comprehensive Treatise*, vol. 4, *Nutrition: Metabolic and Clinical Applications,* ed. R. E. Hodges (New York: Plenum, 1979), p. 102.

Wilkes, E. *Drug Management of Chronic Disease and Other Problems* (London: Faber and Faber, 1982), p. 269.

Wolfe, S. M. and Coley, C. M. *Pills That Don't Work* (New York: Farrar, Straus & Giroux, 1981).

5
NUTRIENT SUPPLEMENTATION

No doubt all nutritional problems could be solved by food, but unless we are so sanguine as to imagine that an optimal diet will in the near future be available for all, it would be well to consider possible strategies to minimize the adverse effects of malnutrition.

DAVID ROWE, M.D.

The days of frank vitamin deficiency in this country are almost extinct. Except for scattered cases found in schizophrenics, hermits, chronic severe alcoholics and other truly unusual situations, the average person gets enough supplementation from cereals and "enriched" grain products so that full-blown cases of beriberi and pellagra are relics of the past.

The RDAs: an outdated gauge

The Recommended Daily Allowances (RDAs) that were set up as nutritional guidelines were designed by looking for clusters of symptoms that fit into disease patterns. The emerging field of preventive medicine, however, makes such guidelines obsolete. But these newer ideas are often dismissed because you can't prove what you don't get.

There are major health problems (other than those caused by severe vitamin deficiency) that are currently recognizable as arising from nutritional deficiencies. However, the cause of these health problems is not being searched out by the average practicing physician. Among them are low-grade deficiency diseases of dietary fiber, macro- and microminerals and essential fatty acids. Deficiencies in any single one of these contribute to less than optimum health. Combined with an excess of antinutrients—refined carbohydrates, hydrogenated fats, chemical pollutants, caffeine, alcohol, tobacco, insecticides, detergents, and so on—even low-grade deficiencies could and do produce nonspecific degenerative diseases. Add to this the already debilitated state of being "sick and in the hospital," and malnutrition is the order of the day.

Every five years or so, the National Academy of Sciences convenes to upgrade the RDAs. In 1985, this group of prestigious scientists disagreed on how much of certain nutrients we require to stay healthy. Perhaps the disagreement stems from our more advanced methods of evaluating information. Or perhaps it is because of a growing awareness that the RDAs may be adequate but not optimal. *Adequate* may not be enough; good health comes from *optimal* nutrition.

Even if you accept the RDAs as guidelines, note this: it

has been demonstrated that to achieve the RDAs from a diet of ordinary store-bought food in most major metropolitan areas of this country, you would have to consume at least 2000 calories a day. Surely that figure must skyrocket for hospital food. *Supplementation is necessary to attain an optimum state of health for most people.*

There are many unknown but very essential nutrient cofactors in food that make it different from supplements. Supplementing does not give license to eat poorly. Supplements simply add those nutrients that should have been in the diet to begin with, or are required in excess because of special need. If we lived on farms in unpolluted environments and could pick and pluck and pull food grown in healthy soil as needed, we would not require supplements.

Assessing the nutrient regimen

Few will disagree that the nutritional needs of patients are not clearly understood by hospital personnel, and that concern for these needs is a very low priority. Since physicians are not trained in nutritional counseling, there is no distinct designation of responsibility for nutrient supplementation. Even if a patient is well enough to eat all the food served in a day, studies show that the levels of many nutrients in hospital food fall below the RDAs, which are already below par for meeting the needs of hospitalized patients.

Although most nurses cannot prescribe the use of supplements (yet), you can ask these questions:

1 Do you take supplements at home?
2 Would you like to continue your supplements in the hospital?

3 If you don't take supplements, would you like guidance in developing a supplement program?

When a patient who is already taking supplements is told that supplementing is "not necessary," the message imparted is that extra vitamins and minerals are not important. This can be undermining. If the answer to the first two questions is yes, you can inform the doctor that the patient would like to continue the home regimen and avoid withdrawal symptoms. Since the doctor now knows that the patient is accustomed to supplements, permission is more than likely.

If the patient is interested in starting a program, you can inform the doctor that you are knowledgeable in this area. This should be accepted as a nursing function. (Doctors already know that nurses help people get better.)

You must remember that any medical regimen requires some behavioral change of the patient. Taking oral supplements is often least difficult, while profound changes in diet are the most difficult. Until you feel comfortable and secure in recommending a nutritional supplement regimen, this chapter can serve as a guide.

If two people are deprived of a specific nutrient, their deficiency symptoms are unlikely to be identical. Symptoms, despite similar causes, are contingent on genetic makeup, age, environment (including stress or lack of it), exercise, drug intake and general health status. Given all these variations, how can it be determined who, if anyone, should take what vitamin or mineral? We believe there is a basic formula from which everyone can benefit, regardless of how healthy or sick that person happens to be. Nutrients which meet specific needs because of biochemical individuality and environmental circumstances should be added.

The basics: a general outline for everyone

A good multi-purpose formula should contain:

Vitamins: A, beta-carotene, thiamin (B1), riboflavin (B2), niacinamide (B3), pantothenic acid, pyridoxine (B6), B12, C (at least 500 milligrams), folic acid, biotin, D (preferably cholecalcipherol), E (in the D-alpha form plus mixed tocopherols)
Amino Acids: cysteine, methionine, and glutamic acid
Lipogenic nutrients: choline and inositol
Minerals: calcium, magnesium, potassium, zinc, copper, manganese, iodine (from kelp), molybdenum, chromium (preferably from yeast), selenium (preferably from yeast)
Additional beneficial nutrients: bioflavonoids, PABA, ascorbyl palmitate (a lipid-soluble vitamin C), octacosanol, garlic, bee pollen, royal jelly, aloe, betaine hydrochloride (to aid absorption)

ABOUT ANTIOXIDANTS

There should no longer be any doubt about the necessity of antioxidants for longevity and avoidance of degenerative disease. Researchers have proved that antioxidants stabilize the all-important membrane functions in every cell of the body. This prevents the submicroscopic damage to the cells themselves, which ultimately leads to impaired cellular function, progressing to tissues and organs and finally to vital functions of the entire body. The mechanism at work is known technically as "free radical pathology." While it may not account for every degenerative problem, it is the major factor in a number of chronic degenerative diseases.

In addition, these antioxidants protect against the conversion of precursors of carcinogenic substances into the actual carcinogen itself. A specific example is the protection that vitamin C affords against the ingested nitrates which are converted in the body to carcinogenic substances known as nitrosamines.

ABOUT MINERALS

Minerals are best absorbed as complexes with amino acids, that is, chelated. Safe levels of individual trace elements can be affected by the amount of other trace minerals present. Indiscriminate ingestion of any mineral supplement is inadvisable because of possible complex interactions.

All trace elements can be toxic, but intake levels must be relatively high. However, intake levels not far above normal can produce subclinical effects. A deficiency or overabundance of the same element can cause the same disease. For example, too much or too little iodine will cause goiter. So you can see the importance of not taking mineral supplements haphazardly, and the advantages of using a well-researched formulation.

Essential fatty acids

Good basic lipid formulas are:

OMEGA-3 LIPID FORMULA

EPA (eicosapentaenoic acid)	540 mg
DHA (docosahexaenoic acid)	360 mg
d-alpha tocopherol	21 mg

OMEGA-6 LIPID FORMULA	
GLA (gamma-linolenic acid) from black currant seed oil (in 250 mg of oil)	40 mg

Essential fatty acids (EFA) are as important as vitamins, minerals and proteins. They form the basic building blocks from which all the body fats (chief energy store), biological membranes (phospholipids and glycolipids) and prostaglandins (hormone-like regulatory substances) are synthesized.

Nonessential fatty acids are those which the body can manufacture. They do not have to come from the food you eat. EFAs, on the other hand, must be in the food supply. However, when there are large amounts of nonessential saturated fatty acids in your diet, they compete with EFAs and suppress their activity. This internal civil war results in the reduction of the important EFAs. Nonessential fatty acids are found in processed saturated fats, such as meat, processed cheese, ersatz ice cream products, nondairy coffee creamers, bakery products, potato chips, crackers, mixes and so on.

Since the average American diet contains such a high rate of nonessential fatty acids, supplementation with EFAs is advisable to help balance the ratio. Because emotional stress depresses the immune system, patients under such stress should be informed about the role of EFAs. It is theorized that because EFAs promote T-lymphocyte activity, this immune system booster has a positive effect on emotions.

ABOUT OMEGA-3 OILS

Omega-3 fatty acids (EPA and DHA) are found only at relatively low levels in the average American diet. Supplements of these fatty acids are usually derived from selected cold water fish from Norwegian or Alaskan waters. The advantages of Omega-3 EFAs came to light in studies of the traditional Eskimo diet, which is very high in protein, fat, cholesterol and retinol (vitamin A), and low in fiber and tocopherols (vitamin E). The traditional Eskimo has low blood cholesterol and an absence of noninfective Western disease, such as cancer, arthritis, diabetes, and others. The fat of Arctic marine animals is the most unsaturated of all animals, and is particularly rich in the Omega-3 oils. There is no doubt that fatty fish can greatly lower blood triglycerides, lower the "bad guy" fractions of cholesterol (LDL and VLDL—low density lipoproteins and very low density lipoproteins), and raise the "good guy" fractions (HDL—high density lipoproteins), as well as decrease platelet aggregation. (Wouldn't it be nice if the physician prescribed herring and mackerel instead of aspirin for patients with platelet aggregation problems!)

Most of these formulas contain an antioxidant (such as vitamin E, d-alpha tocopherol) to ensure stability and potency. Fish oils contain little vitamin E. This is no problem when fresh fish is consumed, but the oils do get rancid easily when extracted from the fish.

ABOUT OMEGA-6 OILS

A most important discovery was the role that polyunsaturated fatty acids play in the production of prostaglandins. Prostaglandins are biological regulators which control many bodily functions. GLA is necessary for the manufacture of prostaglandins, which in turn activate T-lymphocytes, and inhibit smooth muscle proliferation and thrombosis, among other attributes. GLA can only be manufactured in the body through a complex series of metabolic processes.

This function declines with age. In fact, it is impaired in experimental manipulation which accelerates aging and is enhanced in instances of delayed aging; it is also depressed under the stress of illness and hospitalization. Foods rich in saturated fats and cholesterol, foods containing hydrogenated vegetable oils (margarines and cooking oils), diabetes, viral infections and zinc deficiency also block GLA manufacture.

According to current research, hospitalized patients are major candidates for the beneficial effects of GLA supplementation—especially as derived from black currant seed oil, one of the richest sources of GLA. In addition, black currant seed oil provides linoleic and alpha-linolenic acids as well as the rare stearidonic acid.

GLA administration has been found to lower blood pressure and cholesterol, and to cause clinical improvement in patients with scleroderma and alcoholism. These diseases are associated with some features of accelerated aging. The mechanism at work is a blocked enzyme, which can be bypassed by administering GLA directly.

Abnormal proportions of polyunsaturated and saturated fats are found in women with breast cancer. Partial correction has been demonstrated with GLA supplementation, which has also been reported to alleviate breast tenderness. In one research project, six grams of GLA was administered daily to women with fibrocystic disease, with positive results.

Additional supplements

CHLORELLA—THE ONE-CELLED WONDER

The Japanese eat aquatic plants in many forms and in great quantity. They know, for example, that algae are healthful. Algae harbor nutrients in percentages not commonly found in most foods in your local supermarket. A one-celled organism called *chlorella* (chlor for green; ella for small), is among the most popular aquatic plants in Japan (there are many major companies that grow and distribute nothing else). In our country, chlorella has recently been tableted for your convenience.

Chlorella is an independent plant, containing everything it needs to maintain life in its cell. It is a raw, whole food containing chlorophyll, protein, vitamins, minerals, nucleic acids and even polyunsaturated fatty acids. Chlorella has been shown to enhance immune responses and liver function; it also contains antiviral components and cold-reducing properties. It is especially valuable for anyone who is sick and on the mend because of its nucleic acid content.

CARROT-GROWN ACIDOPHILUS

Carrot-grown acidophilus, grown on carrot juice, and called carodophilus, vegedophilus and so on, unloads a few billion acidophilus organisms per gram. Acidophilus bacteria set up housekeeping in your intestine, creating an ecological system that helps the body absorb nutrients and create new ones.

Acidophilus is also available in a milk base. A similar

helpful bacterium (*lactobacillus bulgaricus,* perhaps a second cousin once removed) is found in yogurt, but only in viable yogurt. Not all supermarket yogurts are "live." (Natural food store proprietors can direct you to the "live" yogurt.) Your great-grandmother produced another equally beneficial strain by "clabbering" or souring milk in her kitchen.

Effective dose: one or two capsules after every meal.

Pre- and postoperative priming

Postoperative patients undergo complex and typical changes. Weight loss has been used as a rapid, inexpensive assessment for predicting postoperative complications. But it's not that simple. Only recently have health professionals gained greater appreciation for the benefits of adequate nutrition and appropriate metabolic care prior to and following surgery. It is a fact that patients with low nutritional status stay in the hospital almost twice as long as those whose nutritional status is more normal.

One study with animals demonstrated that the postoperative diet is important for the survival of animals undergoing major and serious surgery. The best postoperative success was achieved with a diet rich in nutrients.

Dr. Howard Bezoza, a nutrition-oriented surgeon from New York City, outlined this plan for patients facing surgery:

- No smoking or coffee for two weeks before surgery. This is to avoid withdrawal from these drugs during surgery, and to encourage good blood vessel flow. Both nicotine and caffeine cause vasoconstriction, which in turn diminishes oxygen that would be brought to the area of surgery.

- Start simple breathing exercises two weeks before surgery to increase oxygenation. Taking long walks may be the easiest way to accomplish this goal.

- Drink lots of water. As estrogen diminishes, the ability to maintain hydration may become somewhat impaired. This is one of the reasons why the skin becomes a little raggedy and wrinkly. A minimum of six glasses a day is necessary.

- The important nutrients in wound healing are:

1 *Zinc.* The definitive cofactor for the ability to cross-link collagen. (In other words, to hold it together.) Collagen is the main supportive protein of skin, tendon, bone, cartilage and connective tissue. It represents approximately 3 percent of total body protein.

2 *Ascorbic acid.* Plays a critical role in wound repair as a cofactor during collagen manufacture.

3 *Sulfur.* Sulfur amino acids are necessary in cross-bonding. (Eggs contain sulfur amino acids.)

It is clear that immune function is highly dependent on the nutritional status of the individual.

- If available, get involved in sauna or whirlpool therapy. Sitting in the steam room and getting massages provides muscular relaxation, and increases the amount of blood flow without muscle use. This, like exercise, helps in the removal of cellular waste products. The ancients gathered in the baths, not so much to be social, but mainly because it made them feel better. They were oxygenating their tissues.

- Following surgery, vitamin E may be used as a topical agent. It is an antioxidant, which means it prevents bacterial growth. It helps stabilize cell membranes, thereby decreasing the incidence of wound breakdown. This helps override excessive scarring.

- Instead of codeine, which is constipating, the aloe vera plant should be used as a superior anesthetic. It may prove to be the best local anesthetic around. Since pure aloe vera is not easy to secure, the best alternative is to buy the plant itself. If it weren't for aloe vera, South American Indians and native American Indians would probably not have survived in the sun. These groups were not dark-complected, and therefore did not have protecting pigment.

Formula regimen for the pill user

For female patients on the Pill, the following are recommended:

- B-complex vitamins, including folate, vitamin B12 and vitamin B6 (organ meats contain these nutrients)
- Brewer's yeast and soybeans (for additional B6)
- Almonds and whole grains (for magnesium)
- Green leafy vegetables (for calcium, magnesium and vitamin C)
- Asparagus and spinach (for additional folate)
- Fermented foods such as tempeh (for additional B12)
- Raw guavas, raw cabbage, raw broccoli and red peppers (for vitamin C)

Bibliography

Beare-Rogers, J. L. "Docosenoic Acids in Dietary Fats." *Progress in Chemical Fats and Other Lipids* 15(1977):29.

Dunbar, J. M., and Stunkard, A. J. "Adherence to Diet and Drug Regimen." In *Nutrition, Lipids, and Coronary Heart Disease*, eds. R. Levy, et al. (New York: Raven Press, 1979).

Kamen, B. and Kamen, S. *In Pursuit of Youth: Everyday Nutrition for Everyone Over 35* (New York: Dodd, Mead & Co., 1984), p. 60.

Brush, M. G. "Efamol in the Treatment of the Premenstrual Syndrome." Special Report, Department of Gynecology, St. Thomas's Hospital Medical School, London, 1981.

Editorial, "Eskimo Diets and Diseases." *Lancet* 1(1983):1139.

Horrobin, D. "Loss of Delta-6-Desaturase Activity as the Key Factor in Aging." *Medical Hypotheses* 7(1981):1211.

Levine, S. "Oxidants, AntiOxidants, and Chemical Hypersensitivities," part 2. *International Journal of Biosocial Research* 4(1983):102.

Rudin, D. Lecture, Orthomolecular Society, Huxley Institute, New York, December 1982.

Sinclair, H. M. "Nutrition and Atherosclerosis." Symposium of the Zoological Society of London, 21(1968):275.

Traitler, H. et al. "Characterization of Gamma-Linolenic Acid in Ribes Seed." *Lipids* 19(1984):923.

6
DISEASE AND NUTRITIONAL SUPPORT

We take medicines that we know very little about, into our bodies that we know even less about, to cure diseases that we don't know anything at all about.

VOLTAIRE

Obviously, life and health are important to every person. They become very important for those who are immediately threatened by disease or death. When disease has taken hold, the immune system is suppressed. Despite overwhelming evidence that suggests nutrients improve immune status, there are still those who consider nutritional intervention as unorthodox and unconventional.

Health care delivery must encourage wellness with nutritional enhancement programs. The benefits that are possible from an improved nutritional environment are mind-boggling. The body has amazing healing powers.

Classifications don't always work

Medical science has been divided in a number of different ways. Sometimes the divisions are more misleading than helpful, especially when using symptoms to label disease. For example, recent studies have shown that coronary arteries in patients diagnosed as having angina pectoris can be completely normal; esophageal problems can cause chest pains that are impossible to differentiate from the pains of angina pectoris. So esophageal pains have been treated with heart medicine. (Not all is lost, however. Nitroglycerin also has a therapeutic effect on esophageal pains.) Another example is the fluoride toxicity that presents with symptoms similar to arthritis. The illustrations are endless.

New information has emerged with advanced technical resources, but this newly acquired knowledge has not always led to more success in preventing or curing disease.

The traditional medical field emphasizes classifications and diagnostic methods. This often creates a disadvantage for therapeutic experiments. The old saying that "an expert is a person who knows more and more about less and less" actually applies here.

Diagnosing disease has become the most important priority for physicians. How can a patient be treated if the physician doesn't know what the patient is suffering from? Too often, diagnosing consumes more of the doctor's time and energy (and the patient's money) than the actual treatment. Many renowned medical philosophers (Goldberger and Williams, among others) have questioned the value of diagnosis. They point out, for example, that even when large groups of people are diagnosed as having the same disease, individual differences are more significant than the similarities.

Goldberg offers the classic example of two people who have ulcers. One is doing shift work and is also having marital problems. The other isn't under either of these stresses. "The difference between the two situations," said Goldberg, "can be greater than between two patients who have different medical diagnoses—for example, arthritis and asthma."

The difficulties are compounded when we consider that autopsies confirm that 30 to 50 percent of the clinicians' diagnoses have been wrong or incomplete.

The wholistic approach

Whether the diagnosis is correct or not, modern medicine does not have "sure" treatments for most diseases. We believe that although diagnoses may differ, treatment for various illnesses or diseases should be largely the same.

Calcium deficiency leads to bone depletion, but there are many enzyme systems which depend on calcium, and every cell in the body—in addition to those of the bone—is affected ultimately by a lack of calcium. In a similar way, deficiencies of essential amino acids lead to generalized problems capable of impairing any and every tissue.

Just as any deficiency of a single nutrient affects every cell in the body, all disorders with a cellular origin can be helped by improving cellular nutrition—regardless of the diagnosis of the disease state. The therapy we suggest includes creating optimal environmental conditions, the most important aspect of which is *diet*. The therapy is similar for different disease states because disease, or health, is based on the cell, which is the unit of life. Every functioning part of our bodies is built of cells. Optimal nutrition that fosters the health of one cell is good for all cells.

This chapter cites noninvasive treatments for many common diseases. The therapies listed come from credible sources, are not dangerous, and have been reported to be helpful. Basically, their value has been to influence the immune system. Although it would have been our preference to eliminate classifications, they are an intrinsic part of today's health care.

The nurse has some authority in a wide variety of health topics, which should include nutrition. If you have little or no influence over the nutritional therapy of a particular patient, you can still inform him or her why they should not consume non-nutritious foods, and encourage foods that are health-promoting.

ARTHRITIS AND NUTRITIONAL SUPPORT

Vitamin D deficiency plays an important role in chronic rheumatoid arthritis. The fact that patients with advanced arthritis rarely leave home compounds the problem; they do not receive much vitamin D from sunlight. A daily supplement of vitamin D is recommended.

If large doses of aspirin are consumed, generous amounts of vitamin C are required. Aspirin depletes vitamin C.

Vitamin B6 (50 to 100 mg daily), plus magnesium and

vitamin C, have been reported to relieve stiffness of the hands.

Certain rheumatoid arthritis-like diseases may be related to an imbalance between zinc and copper. In one study, the use of zinc supplements ranging from 50 to 150 milligrams a day was helpful in reducing symptoms of arthritis.

Dr. William Kaufman, renowned medical researcher, discovered that niacin effectively reverses arthritis. Another well-known London researcher, reports that pantothenic acid (25 to 50 mg daily) has a beneficial effect.

Arthritic symptoms are often related to food allergy. Eliminating allergy-promoting foods is worth a trial run. (See list of the most common allergies later in this chapter.) Overactivation of the mast cell releases inflammation-producing substances that can produce arthritic-like symptoms. This overactivation can come from allergy-producing materials.

Constipation can also lead to the buildup of these immune-sensitizing substances. A high-fiber diet is advisable.

Exercise can have highly beneficial results. The same exercise that produces pain may eventually improve the problem and prevent the joint from "freezing" from nonuse.

Anecdotal reports suggest the use of alfalfa sprouts and fresh cherries for relief of arthritic symptoms.

CANCER AND NUTRITIONAL SUPPORT

It is advisable to reduce the proportion of fat in a cancer patient's diet. The average American diet is comprised of 40 percent fat, which should be cut back to no more than 25 percent. Note that the source of fat is extremely important. Avocados are vastly more nutritious than hamburgers, yet both foods are high in fat. All forms of processed fat are suspected of being cancer promoters. This translates to: no salad dressings; no seeds or nuts that taste bitter (to avoid rancidity); no baked goods; no peanut butter; no ice cream, chips or french fries.

Include vegetables that are especially high in vitamin C and beta-carotene: dark green, orange and deep yellow vegetables and members of the cabbage family. Whole grains (especially brown rice, millet and buckwheat) are excellent choices, as are legumes (peas and beans). Eliminate all pickled and smoked foods, and foods containing chemicals and additives (whenever possible).

Beta-carotene is important in the treatment of lung cancer. Vitamin A may be toxic in doses higher than 20,000 units per day; beta-carotene is not.

Zinc, selenium and manganese are important immune system enhancers. Zinc affects the thymus gland (the master gland of the immune system). Cancer mortality has been correlated with lower levels of dietary selenium intake. Tumors (including mammary tumors) induced by carcinogens have responded to dietary or injected selenium. (Two hundred micrograms daily is recommended for immune protection.) Manganese activates enzymes that are protective. (The recommended dose is between 5 and 20 milligrams daily. Brussels sprouts and cabbage contain high levels of selenium and manganese.)

Vitamins C and E, when used together, have been shown to improve the management of some tumors by inhibiting cancer growth and reducing the side effects of chemotherapy.

B vitamins improve appetite.

The antibiotic activity of cultured products like acidophilus and viable yogurt helps inhibit the growth of harmful bacteria and reduces the risk of colon cancer.

Since radiation therapy alters the sense of taste and smell, remember that patients with a distorted sense of smell often find cold foods more acceptable than hot foods.

Glucose intolerance is frequently observed in cancer patients. This may blunt sensations of hunger. To help appetite, foods should be of the highest quality in terms of appearance.

Malabsorption is a concomitant of both radiation and chemotherapy. Abdominal radiation blunts the intestinal villi, leading to a decrease in absorptive surfaces. Absorption aids should be employed (acidophilus, digestive enzymes, and so on).

Most patients receiving chemotherapy experience nausea and vomiting at the time or shortly after the agent is administered. Chemotherapy should not be given for at least two hours before or two hours after a meal.

Weight loss is common for the majority of cancer patients, probably because cancer cells use energy and nutrients for growth. Careful attention to the nutritional needs of cancer patients is essential. It is easier for the patient to take supplements than to eat foods when there is no appetite. This is not to say that eating should not be encouraged, but you should not make the patient feel pressured to eat. Understanding and sensitivity are paramount, even though you know that well-nourished patients have a more positive response to therapy than malnourished patients.

HEART DISEASE AND NUTRITION

Elevated blood cholesterol, cholesterol deposits in the skin and similar deposits in the arteries to the legs that obstruct blood flow have been treated successfully with extremely large doses of niacin.

Many patients with high blood pressure also have elevated levels of cadmium. Sources of cadmium are cigarette smoke, automobile exhaust, refined foods and soft or acidic drinking water. Antioxidants help eliminate toxins like cadmium. Zinc is a known antagonist of cadmium.

Moderate increases in natural foods containing cholesterol are *not* related to increased risk of heart disease. Increased blood cholesterol usually results from stress and the consumption of processed fat, as well as other factors that encourage the body to increase its synthesis. Although egg yolks (commonly blamed for increasing cholesterol levels) contain cholesterol, they also contain lecithin. Lecithin emulsifies cholesterol and other fats. The egg is one of the most biologically digestible and useful proteins. (And it is also inexpensive.) Eggs should be soft-boiled for maximum benefit.

Beans and peas also lower blood cholesterol. The cholesterol-lowering effect of dried peas and beans may be attributable in part to the action of the lecithin they contain.

A meat-free diet, which decreases the amount of fat ingested, can lower blood cholesterol and help prevent arteriosclerosis. Diets high in animal protein and low in vitamin B6 place the patient at risk for coronary artery disease. A low-fat diet is not only preventive, but can also be therapeutic. It can facilitate the resorption, or uptake, of existing plaque, and may provide a dietary alternative to surgery. A good alternative to animal protein is vegetable protein, which has been found in experiments with animals to protect in some way against arteriosclerosis when compared with animal protein.

Consumption of sugar, salt, processed fats and hydrogenated oils should be avoided.

Omega-3 fatty acids (eicosapentaenoic and docosahexaenoic acids) are highly recommended. These essential fatty acids provide the material from which the body manufactures a substance which prevents platelets from sticking together in the arterial system. If the patient has an appetite, cold water deep-sea fish should be suggested. (The patient should be encouraged to eat the skin, where these essential fatty acids are found.) If appetite is limited, a supplement of these substances as recommended in Chapter 5 is advisable.

Platelet aggregation is also inhibited by onions and garlic. The use of nutritional agents to reduce platelet aggregation, as contrasted to aspirin, is superior. Aspirin increases bleeding time. Garlic or cod-liver oil do not.

Insufficient calcium absorption has been related to high blood pressure. Note that calcium *intake* is not necessarily the most significant factor. (See the section on osteoporosis in this chapter for details on improving calcium absorption.) Silicon-, vitamin D3- and magnesium-deficient diets are associated with impaired heart function. These are also discussed in the section on bone health.

If the patient is on diuretics, potassium deficiency may be a problem. Potassium abounds in green leafy vegetables and sunflower seeds. Since table salt (sodium) competes with potassium, salt should be eliminated. There is enough sodium in natural foods to supply the body's needs. Salt can actually increase the size of the heart, and place a strain on the heart muscle.

It has also been demonstrated that a soybean-rich diet is an effective regimen for a significant reduction in blood cholesterol. Two amino acids that are important in the control of the body's ability to manufacture cholesterol are lysine and arginine.

Test animals who had atherosclerosis were fed a diet enriched with alfalfa. The results were a reduction in blood cholesterol and a regression of atherosclerotic plaques.

The use of a low-saturated fat diet supplemented with large amounts of polyunsaturated fat (such as GLA from black currant seed oil), also lowers cholesterol.

Coffee and black tea have been associated with cardiovascular disease.

Vitamin C reduces the cholesterol of patients who have elevated levels. Marked decreases have been shown with 500 milligrams of vitamin C for people whose levels were above 300 mg percent.

Chromium has been shown to increase HDL. The effective dose is 200 micrograms per day. Vitamin E, at 600 units a day, was also found to increase HDL cholesterol levels.

Carnitine, a naturally occurring amino acid, significantly reduces blood triglycerides when administered in 400 milligram doses, three times daily. Carnitine is effective because it helps in the metabolic process whereby fats are converted to energy.

INFECTIONS AND NUTRITION

Catabolic responses occur in all infectious illnesses, regardless of the agent or the presence of symptoms. Even subclinical or silent infections induce stress responses, with increased nitrogen excretion in the urine.

Nutrients often found lacking in those prone to infectious disease are folic acid, vitamin C, pyridoxine, zinc and magnesium.

Sequestration of nutrients occurs during an infectious process, rendering a nutrient useless for normal metabolic processes. For example, sodium and iron are essentially lost to the body at this time. With sodium sequestration, there may be fluid overloading, whereas the sequestration of iron may lead to anemia.

Most patients who have infections are encouraged to drink "lots of fluids," which often translates to "lots of juice or soda pop." Glucose synthesis is accelerated during the infectious process, and so fluids should be nonsugar drinks, herbal teas, filtered or bottled water or broth made with such water.

A very effective therapy for infection is a concentrated form of lactobacillus acidophilus. (Are we beginning to sound like a broken record?)

BLOOD GLUCOSE AND NUTRITION

Pectin has been shown to slow the gastric release of ingested food, especially sugars. So blood sugar might rise more slowly, resulting in a lower insulin response. Fiber-free substances such as apple juice produce higher insulin levels than do equicaloric quantities of whole apples. Diabetics have demonstrated lower blood sugar levels after consuming meals containing pectin. Perhaps pectin improves diabetic control by reducing the absorption rate of sugar.

Diets high in complex carbohydrates and low in fats always improve glucose tolerance. At the same time they decrease cholesterol levels; thus, this kind of diet should be used for diabetic management. Since diabetics are particularly susceptible to atherosclerosis and its complications, it seems prudent, on the basis of present information, for such patients to consume a diet that favors the reduction of cholesterol and triglyceride blood levels.

For patients with diabetes and hypoglycemia, well-spaced, moderate-sized feedings are preferable to large ones. Simple, concentrated carbohydrates such as sucrose should be avoided. Diabetics who cannot handle rapid alterations in blood sugar should avoid carbohydrates that induce rapid swings in blood sugar.

In the diabetic patient, the conversion from carotene to vitamin A may be impaired. Adequate dietary sources of vitamin A should be available. Liver, eggs and cod-liver oil are the best sources.

Patients with poorly controlled diabetes usually develop deficits of water, sodium, potassium and chloride. This is especially true when diuresis or excessive sweating occurs.

Chromium, a glucose-tolerance factor, is involved with glucose tolerance for many people. Unfortunately, this nutrient is often deficient in Western diets. The body content of chromium decreases with age here, while in Eastern countries, where natural, unprocessed foods are eaten, chromium content remains constant. Chromium is easily lost in the milling of grains and the processing of foods. Chromium-containing foods with biologically active chromium are brewer's yeast, black pepper, liver, whole wheatberries and mushrooms. Brewer's yeast is the best source. Caution: if the patient has been receiving high levels of insulin for some time, the administration of large amounts of yeast too quickly may produce a rebound effect by overstimulation. Brewer's yeast should be introduced gradually into the diet and blood glucose should be monitored carefully in the diabetic patient.

Inositol (500 milligrams twice daily) has helped diabetic patients who have had peripheral nerve damage. In these patients, manganese content of the blood is often half that of normal people. Manganese deficiency impairs glucose metabolism.

Alcohol causes an overstimulation of insulin output, which

accentuates the reactive hypoglycemia that follows glucose loading.

As suggested in the heart disease section above, a low-saturated fat diet supplemented with large amounts of polyunsaturated fat (such as GLA from black currant seed oil), lowers cholesterol. The dietary treatment of hyperlipidemia is essential in patients with diabetes mellitus.

Between-meal snacks, including a small meal before bedtime, are often essential for the diabetic. Those who eat three meals or less per day are significantly more obese, have higher serum cholesterol levels, and diminished glucose tolerance. Frequent feedings, avoiding large evening meals, are far less detrimental to the diabetic. Insulin-dependent diabetics must eat multiple meals to avoid hypoglycemia. Periods of feast or famine must be avoided.

Exercise is another positive therapeutic tool that can be used to sensitize tissues to insulin and increase insulin binding.

It is not possible to control diabetes unless diet therapy is optimal. When caring for a diabetic, the nurse must be well informed and persistent. There is a marked decrease in the triglyceride levels in people who are given nutritional counseling as compared to those who are not advised about diet. So don't hesitate to use your knowledge and educate.

In summary, high-fiber diets lower blood sugar, decrease glycosuria, decrease insulin needs and increase tissue sensitivity to insulin. Whenever feasible, natural foods containing unrefined carbohydrate with fiber should be substituted for highly refined carbohydrates, which are low in fiber.

OSTEOPOROSIS (AND OTHER BONE DISEASES) AND NUTRITION

Accompanying the loss of ovarian function for many women is osteoporosis. Care of women with hip fractures from osteoporosis has become a public health issue which possibly suggests a lack of patient education regarding health maintenance. Nurses can play a key role in caring for osteoporosis patients by knowing what causes the disease. A broad understanding of patient management, including the important area of nutrition education and health maintenance is invaluable.

The modeling and remodeling of bone involves the interaction of organs, hormones and minerals. Any nutritional defect that affects the transport protein system, endocrine function, liver function, kidney function or protein or collagen manufacture will affect bone metabolism. Diabetes, thyrotoxicosis (overactive thyroid) or any disease requiring extended bed rest causes rapid excretion of calcium, and consequently osteoporosis.

People with Crohn's disease often have bone disease. These people have severe malabsorption problems, including losses of vitamin D.

A large variety of drugs used in the treatment of different diseases contributes to osteoporosis. Chronic administration of glucocorticoids may produce osteoporosis. These drugs have been shown to decrease ascorbic acid levels in test animals. Patients on long-term dilantin and phenobarbital treatment for epilepsy may also develop bone disease.

Even if calcium intake is adequate, calcium *absorption* may be reduced and calcium balance may be negative—especially if the patient is deficient in vitamin D.

You can see how important calcium absorption is. Guidelines follow for helping patients understand the processes involved in calcium absorption. Patients should:

Take a brief sunbath daily, if possible. The sun is the best source of vitamin D. The patient need only expose a small amount of bare skin for half an hour during the middle of the day.

Consume vitamin D-containing foods and take cod-liver oil to augment vitamin D supplies. (Toxicity rarely occurs from a natural form of vitamin D, though it can occur when given in isolated form.) If a fresh source of cod-liver oil is unavailable, or the patient cannot tolerate its taste, 400 IU in supplemental form presents no risk of toxicity.

Eat organ meats. For proper vitamin D metabolism, you need a healthy liver and healthy kidneys to convert the vitamin to its active, hormonal form. Although organ meat is not the economical food it used to be, it's still a bargain.

Take antioxidants to help the liver function optimally. An antioxidant is a substance that prevents oxygen deterioration. Antioxidants available in supplemental form are vitamins A, C and E, plus B1 and B2; beta-carotene, inositol, lecithin, zinc, and selenium. The amino acids found in eggs are also antioxidants.

Legumes (any kind of peas, beans or lentils) are foods that work as antioxidants. They help the body to detoxify—to get rid of unwanted toxins.

Eat fish from deep ocean waters.

Consume calcium, both in food and supplemental form. Four hundred to 800 milligrams of calcium is a good preventive dose. Calcium-containing foods are: green vegetables like turnip greens, mustard greens, broccoli and kale (use steamer and cook lightly to preserve nutrients); legumes and nuts; shellfish; whole grain cereal products (60 percent of calcium in wheat is lost in refining of flour); sardines and other small fish in which bones are eaten.

Tofu is a high-calcium food. A serving of 3½ ounces

contains 128 milligrams of calcium. Not only is tofu low in fat, but it has a respectable amount of protein, other minerals and B vitamins too.

Use supplements like chlorella and ginseng to aid in liver detoxification. (Chlorella was discussed in detail in Chapter 5.) Ginseng is a root that is frequently used in traditional herbal medicine of the Far East. It is, in fact, one of the most frequently used herbs in traditional herbal medicine because of its long history of success. Ginseng also has an effect on the adrenal glands. These glands are responsible for estrogen manufacture after menopause. Keeping adrenal glands functioning at optimal levels is an excellent way to keep bones healthy.

Stay away from sugar. Refined sugar inhibits calcium absorption. Refined sugar alters insulin metabolism, which in turn affects calcium metabolism. In addition, sugar requires vitamin B6 in order to be metabolized. Vitamin B6 plays a role in magnesium pathways, which in turn affects bone. Furthermore, vitamin B6 helps regulate estrogen levels.

Avoid processed fatty acids, found in margarine and other processed foods. Essential fatty acids affect calcium absorption.

Gamma-linolenic acid is an important supplement, especially as derived from black currant seed oil. Most people have difficulty converting polyunsaturated oils to this activated form (GLA). Without the conversion, the body cannot manufacture prostaglandins. Prostaglandins are essential to bone health.

Exercise, deep breathing and some yoga should be lifetime habits. Teach your patients some of these techniques. (Stretching stimulates osteoblasts, the cells which form bone.)

Using additional supplements to cover all bases is a good idea. Follow the recommendations outlined in Chapter 5.

If you think milk should have been added to this list, read carefully: *milk is not a recommended beverage or food, even for women at risk for osteoporosis.* A significant amount of current research shows that milk is not an optimal or even desirable food for many reasons. Lactose intolerance (discussed elsewhere)—even if subclinical—can be a problem; and pasteurization destroys nutrients and homogenization alters fat molecules. Low-fat or skim milk is even more processed and less nutritious.

BURNS AND NUTRITION

Sufficient calorie intake is important for burn patients, especially if the burns are serious. This is necessary because of the characteristic tissue catabolism, particularly if there is superimposed infection and fever. But hospitals depend heavily on refined carbohydrates for calories, even though such foods are devoid of vitamins and minerals. (Examples are ice cream, jello and soda pop.) And read the labels on the canned liquids used in tube feedings and assess for yourself how complete a diet that appears to be.

Given our knowledge about nutrient-deficient refined foods, and the inclination of traditional caregivers to equate high calories with highly refined foods, what price must burn patients pay by following requests to eat lots of sugar?

Vitamin C (at least one to two grams daily) should be given orally. This should be continued to counteract the lowering of serum ascorbic acid values which usually accompanies major burns, and to promote wound healing. Vitamin

C helps maintain normal matrixes of cartilage, dentine and bone.

Complete multivitamin supplementation (with emphasis on the B complex) in therapeutic doses is essential. Thiamin is necessary for the metabolism of carbohydrate; the recommended requirement is based on the daily caloric intake. Since the latter is increased in burned patients, the B vitamins should also be increased proportionately. The same holds true for the intake of vitamins A and D. Since an excess of vitamins A and D cannot be excreted, care must be taken not to overdose. Even though it is doubtful that a fat-soluble vitamin toxicity would develop during the usual duration of the postburn course, a natural supplement such as cod-liver oil is advisable.

The pain from major burns requires the use of either narcotics or some form of sedation. All of these agents inhibit appetite, and they sometimes induce nausea and constipation. Side effects which involve appetite and food intake should be kept in mind and noted.

Some clinicians recommend the use of 100 milligrams of pyridoxine daily (by mouth, in divided doses).

A high-protein diet is appropriate to replace the extensive protein loss through the exudate at the burn site. However, an excessive intake of protein and sodium without adequate fluid intake can lead to dehydration, hypernatremia and an elevated BUN level. This is particularly hazardous for older patients with impaired renal function. Therefore, when a tube feeding for an older patient provides more than 1½ to 2 grams of protein per kilogram of body weight per day, the fluid intake and output should be carefully measured and recorded daily, and the intake of protein in grams per kilogram of body weight should also be recorded daily on the patient's chart. Too concentrated a feeding can also result if the commercial products that come in powdered or concentrated form are not reconstituted according to the manufacturer's directions.

If watery diarrhea occurs in a patient receiving a tube feeding that has been administered correctly, it may be due to the carbohydrate content. The lactose in excessive amounts of milk may cause diarrhea in some patients. In this case a feeding that is lactose-free should be used.

The fluids administered via IV are medical orders, but the nurse can choose and monitor oral fluids. And you should think *nutrition,* not just fluids.

Wound healing proceeds more satisfactorily and the hazards of infection are lessened when nutritional status is maintained. Nutritional requirements are greater during the strongly catabolic phase than they are during late convalescence. If the patient is malnourished at the time of injury, more protein is required for equilibrium.

When the patient feels well enough to eat, dietary protein must be of good quality and must contain all of the essential amino acids. For the vegetarian, the addition of sesame seeds is recommended as an addition to grains and salads. Sesame seeds contain the amino acids which are in short supply in most plant foods. Note that it is most important to use sesame seeds which have been mechanically hulled. Most brands on the market are chemically hulled, and the chemicals used are absorbed by the seed, making it detrimental rather than beneficial to health. Mechanically hulled seeds have a tiny black umbilicus visible, which is missing on the chemically hulled product.

If iron deficiency becomes a problem in the burned patient, vitamin C supplementation is essential. Vitamin C potentiates iron absorption.

The precise requirement for zinc in the burned patient

has not been established, but studies indicate that the amount needed is in excess of the usual quantity recommended for zinc equilibrium. A deficit of zinc may develop shortly after the burn occurs, often persisting for two or three months after injury.

Deficiencies of vitamin B-complex and vitamin A cause delayed wound healing.

It is obvious that burn care requires a high staff-to-patient ratio. Hospital budgets that support this care are mandatory.

ALCOHOLISM, DRUG ABUSE AND NUTRITION

Many nurses have cared for patients with drug abuse problems, most commonly alcohol and cocaine abuse. These patients may have health problems directly related to the drug abuse, but not identified by their physician. In many cases the physician is "the last to know." These same patients may choose not to deal with the drug abuse, which is, of course, their choice.

These patients remain, however, a high-risk population for malnutrition. If nurses paid as much attention to nutrients as to medications that subvert delirium tremens, progress in the course of treatment could improve. Without diagnosing a condition, the nurse could identify the drug consumption pattern to the physician, and note signs of nutrient deficiency which may be related to the drug consumption. (Some surgeons realize that the alcoholic requires more magnesium and vitamins.)

CONSTIPATION AND NUTRITION

If there is one health condition that nurses can make a significant difference in, it must be constipation. The nurse sees how patients eat and move, and is in the best position to discuss "usual" and "normal" with the patient. A patient may tell you that it is normal for him to have two bowel movements a week. You have to define *usual* as compared with *normal*.

Improper diet is one of the main causes of constipation. Reduced activity of the hospitalized patient may compound the problem.

These substances contribute to constipation:

1 Over-refined and starchy foods (white bread, white rice, bakery products, etc.

2 Hard-boiled eggs, cheese, meat, boiled milk

3 Hot drinks

4 Foods containing tannin (red wine, tea, cocoa, etc.)

5 Cloves

These foods help to eradicate constipation:

1 Foods that absorb moisture readily (celery, radishes, carrots, lettuce)

2 Foods that are slightly laxative (raw figs, raw spinach, strawberries, sesame seeds, watermelon)

3 Lots of fluids

4 Herbs and other high-nutrient foods
   a garlic (prescribed for constipation by Hippocrates)
   b chlorella, an aquatic plant supplement
   c dandelion leaf tea
   d flax seeds

e brewer's yeast
f rice polishings
5 High-fiber foods such as vegetables and whole-grain cereals

Here are two recipes that are very effective (perhaps they could be prepared by the patient's family):

1 Dried prunes soaked overnight in water with lemon juice.

2 A blend of 1 tablespoon of pumpkin seeds, 2 ounces of sesame seeds, 1 cup of soaked raisins. Add enough warm water to make 1 quart: sip through the day.

ALLERGY AND NUTRITION

Many patients are sensitive to the very food they love the most and therefore eat most frequently. Reactions tend to be dose- and frequency-related on an individual basis. A fraction of a drop of cow's milk may cause a reaction in one person, whereas it may take a quart of milk to induce symptoms in another. Nor are reactions always immediate. They could present themselves in fifteen minutes, or a day or two later.

It is essential to be free of food sensitivities if nutrients are to be properly assimilated. Note the percentage of frequency of the twelve most common food allergens found in one thousand food-allergic people:

Food	Number of People with Allergy (in 1000)
Milk	679
Chocolate, cola	400
Corn	302
Citrus	272

Food	Number of People with Allergy (in 1000)
Non-fertile eggs	259
Legumes	229
Tomato	133
Wheat	118
Apple	75
Cinnamon	71
Rice	65
Food coloring	64

Note the difference between the number of people sensitive to milk and to any other food.

WOMEN'S HEALTH CARE

Now that you have been introduced (or reintroduced) to the role that nutrition plays in health and illness, and your consciousness is raised, look at the literature and its relation to women's health. Menstrual distress, premenstrual syndrome, breastfeeding and *Candida* infections are all conditions for which there are specific nutritional interventions. Stretch marks can be prevented and the effects of aging can be reduced.

We are all advised to avoid charlatans, quacks, quick remedies, and anything else relating to health that is nonconventional, i.e. nonmedical. Nutritional medicine is sometimes considered "far out." At the same time, we nurses faithfully dispense drugs as we line up our patients for invasive treatments, with known but often not-discussed serious side effects. Very often, not enough good research has supported these interventions.

This is not a defense for nutrition intervention. Rather, we want you to know that respected scientists and researchers are involved in nutrition research. *Their evidence is solid.*

What would the physician's response be if asked for scientific evidence for procedures or medications? (This is the question they ask nurses when nutrition intervention is suggested.)

The nurse's opportunity to enhance nutrition and encourage the consumption of specific nutrients in the hospital may seem dismal. But we are talking about incremental change. Now that you are more aware of how essential nutrition is to health and healing, you can start (or continue further with) the process of change. We are not suggesting that nutrition change is easy. Nor is it something that your colleagues will embrace tomorrow. We are addressing you, the professional nurse, whose priorities are commitment and effort. You know you can and do make a difference.

Every physician and nurse should be reminded that nutritional deficiency is the commonest cause of secondary impairment of immunocompetence.

Bibliography

Abraham, J. "Management of the Immunocompromised Host." *Medical Clinic of North America* 68(1984): 617.

Burton, B. T. *Human Nutrition* (New York: McGraw-Hill, 1976).

Chandra, R. K. and Newberne, P. M. *Nutrition and Infection: Mechanisms and Interactions* (New York: Plenum Press, 1977).

Friedman, G. J. "Diet in the Treatment of Diabetes Mellitus." In *Modern Nutrition in Health and Disease*, eds. R. S. Goodhart and M. E. Shils (Philadelphia: Lea & Febiger, 1978).

Gray, G. M. and Fogel, M. R. "Nutritional Aspects of Dietary Carbohydrates." In *Modern Nutrition in Health and Disease.*

Handy, L. C. "Nursing Management of the Woman with Osteoporosis." *Journal of Obstetrics and Gynecology* 14(1985):107.

Jarrett, R. J. *Nutrition and Disease* (Baltimore: University Park Press, 1979).

Kamen, B. and Kamen, S. *Osteoporosis: What It Is, How to Stop It, How to Prevent It* (New York: Pinnacle, 1984; St. Martin's Press, 1986).

Littleton, E. M. "The Nutrition Care Profile: An Aid to Delivery of Quality Nutrition Care in a Small Community Hospital." *Journal of the American Dietetic Association* 84(1984):1468.

Lutton, M. S. et al. "Levels of Patient Nutrition Care for Use in Clinical Decision Making." *Journal of the American Dietetic Association* 85(1985):849.

Orr, J. W. and Shingleton, H. M. "Importance of Nutritional Assessment and Support in Surgical and Cancer Patients." *Journal of Reproductive Medicine* 29(1984):635.

Pfeiffer, C. *Mental and Elemental Nutrients: a Physician's Guide to Nutrition and Health Care* (New Canaan, Conn: Keats Publishing, 1975).

Ruberg, R. L. "Role of Nutrition in Wound Healing." *Surgical Clinic of North America* 64(1984):705.

Spallholz, J. E. "Anti-Inflammatory, Immunologic and Carcinostatic Attributes of Selenium in Experimental Animals." In *Advances in Experimental Medicine and Biology,* vol. 135, *Diet and Resistance to Disease,* eds. M. Phillips, and A. Baetz (New York: Plenum Press, 1980).

Todd, E. A. et al. "What Do Patients Eat in Hospital?" *Human Nutrition: Applied Nutrition* 38(1984):294.

Vitale, J. J. "Therapy and Nutritional Support." In *Nutritional Support of Medical Practice,* eds. Schneider et al. (New York: Harper & Row, 1977).

Weyant, H. K. "Go For It." *American Journal of Nursing* 85(1985):850.

7

STRESS AND NUTRITION

When we feel we are under stress, the body mirrors that stress through change in its own health status.

JEFFREY BLAND, PH.D.

A friend of ours told us that when he was a child, his mother scolded him when he cried at the dinner table. The reprimand, explained his mom, had nothing to do with her annoyance at his behavior. "You see," she would say, "when you shed tears while eating, food turns to poison."

It wasn't until our friend became a physician that he learned that digestion does indeed start in one's head. There is an intimate relationship between emotional stress and gastrointestinal malabsorption.

Our personal file on foods grows larger day by day—a file that includes articles detailing just how the impoverished quality of our food (plus the commercial processing it undergoes) is responsible for nutrient depletion. When confronted with pressures, this fault in the foodways of our country places our population at an even higher risk of disease. Combining the intake of "plastic" foods with emotional stress creates a negative effect that is geometrically cumulative. Foods of the high-tech late twentieth century are poor sources for nutrients compared with more natural foods.

We believe every nurse should understand stress mechanisms and how they work. A hospital contains a higher percentage of people under stress than almost any other facility.

Unpleasant images and what your brain does with them

Stress begins its destructive action at the level of the midbrain. A disagreement with either a coworker or supervisor may be upsetting. The image of the altercation travels from the cortex (the outer layer of gray matter in your brain which receives sensory stimuli) to the brain's deeper structures. One of the most important of these deep structures is the hypothalamus, which works like the dispatching station of a telecommunications center. Once it receives the message of an uncomfortable or dangerous situation, it sends stimulating impulses to its entire territory. One of the reactions which then ensues is the production of adrenalin. How many times have you heard and used the expression, "My adrenalin was flowing," a statement denoting excitation. But that's just the tip of the iceberg. The hypothalamus has been considered the possible primary site where the onset of aging is triggered.

The might of the hypothalamus puts the nineteenth-century British Empire to shame. The hypothalamus is in command of activating, empowering and integrating the autonomic mechanisms (those which are self-controlled and which function without conscious effort). These include endocrine activities and many other functions such as fluid regulation, body temperature control, sleep patterns and even food intake.

The hypothalamus is top kingpin of the brain's relay setup. And it alerts all of you to unpleasant or threatening situations. That's the stress effect. Your entire body reacts, and does so with the speed of an electronic messenger.

Of special concern are the functions that occur automatically in the large organs—contractions of the heart, the movement of the gut, the secretion of digestive enzymes and the process of perspiring, to name but a few. All of this happens without mental or physical awareness, in response to events that are being experienced. Any episode may be pleasing or displeasing, and the body responds accordingly.

To review some physiology, this base of operations controlling the body without conscious dictate is divided into two networks called sympathetic and parasympathetic autonomic nervous systems. As you know, an important distinction between these two branches is that the sympathetic is stimulated during times of stress; the parasympathetic regulates, among many other physiological processes, restorative or peaceful functions, including the secretion of gastrointestinal enzymes.

The interpretation of circumstances signals the command for either (but not both) of these systems to prevail. For example, if you are sitting quietly at home reading a delightful novel and listening to a beautiful rendition of Beethoven's Ninth Symphony, your parasympathetic system is operating. If lightning suddenly strikes a tree outside your window, your sympathetic system takes over. You feel the stress effect immediately.

A serious problem develops when you are repeatedly faced with stressors. And herein lies the problem: hospital patients experience many stressors, including multiple staff caregivers, different food, different room environment, different bathroom, fluorescent lighting, separation from loved ones, noise, multiple invasive treatments and medication. These events activate the same stress mechanisms as that bolt of lightning.

When distressing events occur often enough, a person is in a constant state of "high arousal," which is independent of the stimulus. In other words, the sympathetic system becomes the master even during peaceful times. People with this condition have elevated muscle tension and body movement. You have undoubtedly seen the ill-at-ease child twirling hair; the teenager repeatedly tapping a foot; the adult poking with a pencil. These people often lose the ability to shift into the parasympathetic, or calm, mode of behavior—even when they should be free of tension. And so it is with hospitalized patients.

You can see what a vicious cycle this becomes: the muscle tension propagates more stimuli for the sympathetic system. All this "over-firing" is at the expense of the central nervous system; it is often referred to as the burn-out syndrome. The consequences can even modify brain function.

Philosophers refer to the twentieth century as the Age of Uncertainty, the Age of Anxiety, the Age of Rapid Change and even Future Shock—these writers maintain that our perception of external events has become more threatening. The hypothalamus is sending messages of "war" to internal organs with increasing frequency. However, our physiology is still the physiology of the caveperson. We have not evolved with the kind of efficiency that allows differentiation between a mugger going after us with a knife and symbolic threatening situations such as the displeasure, anxiety and trauma of the hospital.

The physiology of the caveperson was geared to very basic functions for survival. Gathering food, reproduction and protecting the herd were prime objectives. The search for food often occurred when supplies were completely diminished. It is unlikely that prehistoric man-of-the-house (cave?) commenced his quest with a meal in his stomach.

As it happens, the first thing that is disrupted during a stressful situation is the ability to digest food and consequently extract nutrients (vitamins and minerals) from it. This is because the stimulus that the hypothalamus perceives as threatening through that figure of authority on the brain, has sent stress messages to internal organs. Since these organs are not essential for immediate survival, blood is diverted from them to the large muscles of the arms and legs—so important in the "fight or flight" mechanism. The body requires a lot of blood in its vessels to run or to fight as the message races through the body, organs squeeze out blood. The spleen (which is the greatest reservoir of blood), liver and kidneys are all involved. The heart rate is also increased and more effective. The body is prepared for activity, *and all digestive functions cease.* (This explains the diarrhea that some people experience following a stressful event. When the system returns to normal, the body has to deal with undigested food.)

There is a fascinating stress/digestion connection because of the constant delicate balance between the sympathetic and parasympathetic systems—the two networks controlled by the hypothalamus. The sympathetic system triggers production of adrenalin. Again, adrenalin means excitation. The parasympathetic system, on the other hand, is responsible for production of acetylcholine, which produces the relaxation response. When imbalances exist between these two chemicals, it is not possible to secrete the gastrointestinal juices necessary for proper digestion. It has even been proposed that the terms sympathetic and parasympathetic be replaced by adrenergic (meaning stimulated, activated or transmitted by adrenalin) and cholinergic (meaning stimulated, activated or transmitted by choline).

Although our ancestors were certainly not cognizant of these fine physiological patterns, their empirical observations and common sense suggested practices that helped them survive with greater ease. At times of distress, Grandma discouraged heavy meals rich in foods that required a great deal of enzymes for digestion. Grandma would certainly discourage such a meal for any family member headed for the hospital.

When the lion lies down with the lamb

When your world is at peace, macronutrients—proteins, fats and carbohydrates—are used to rebuild tissues and provide energy. Very simply, this is how it works:

1. Amino acids are broken down from the protein consumed, and are reassembled into *human* protein, as expressed or conditioned by genetic code. The body takes something else and converts it into *you*.

2. Glucose, not to be confused with refined sugar, is the most immediate source of energy. The brain is its greatest utilizer. Physiologically speaking, glucose is the fastest and most economical source of energy. You know how you feel after you have eaten something sweet. The glucose not needed for energy at the moment is stored mostly as glycogen, or animal sugar. This is meant to be a reserve for times of famine.

3. Fatty acids also enter into the burner for energy. If they are underutilized, the excess fatty acids are also stored as reserves, in the form of fatty deposits known as adipose tissue. These deposits are very hard to dispose of.

Each cell is in essence a laboratory in which all of these events occur. But the stress response shuts down the digestive process responsible for the conversions. The proteins, fats and carbohydrates of which food is composed may simply not break down when the hypothalamus receives unpleasant images. If your patient is not in a relaxed position when eating, he or she will not be able to properly extract:

1 amino acids from protein,
2 glucose from carbohydrates and
3 fatty acids and glycerol from fats.

The very same food that can nourish and nurture now becomes a burden. And an important, often overlooked fact is that the same stress that curtails food breakdown also puts the skids under nutrient supplements! *If you are not absorbing nutrients from food, the chances are you are not absorbing nutrients contained in a tablet or capsule.*

Disruption is not limited to digestion

Hans Selye, renowned for his theories on stress, discusses resistance to disease:

> By *general resistance* I mean the ability to remain healthy—or at least alive—during intense stress caused nonspecifically by various agents . . .
>
> Among newborn infants of foreign women employed in Germany as "guest workers" during an economic boom period, the malformation rate was unusually high, and this has been ascribed to the stressor effect of relocation into an unusual environment.
>
> In guinea pigs and mice exposed to heat during certain stages of pregnancy, embryonic mortality and malformations—particularly brain damage—were often detectable. Various malformations of the brain have also been reported in the offspring of pregnant mice kept under extremely crowded conditions.
>
> *Aging* itself—and particularly premature aging—is, in a sense, due to the constant, and eventually exhausting, stresses of life.

Hans Selye's comments support the view that stress disrupts physiological processes, and thus may be the villain in many degenerative diseases as well as a cause of abnormalities.

Here are findings of a few studies which outline other disturbances induced by stress:

- Endorphins are substances produced in the brain. They are self-made morphine, the built-in mechanism for easing pain. Endorphins are believed to have a profound effect on mood, which correlates with a sense of wellbeing. In response to mild stress, the levels of endorphins in test animals fall significantly. This is one reason that patients feel more pain when under stress.

- Under certain conditions, the body releases its own opiates (again, pain-relieving substances). These secretions increase at times of stress, but they inhibit intestinal secretions necessary for digestion. This is why patients are more prone to digestive disorders when under stress.

- Collagen is a fibrous protein found in connective tissue, bone and cartilage. There is a relationship between the production of this kind of protein in the arteries and the atherosclerotic process. Stress promotes the manufacture of collagen. This is one connection between stress and heart disease.

- When under stress, hormones are secreted which reduce the efficacy of the white blood cells or T-cells, the body's soldier cells. T-cells are involved in defense against disease. This is why stress reduces immunity to infection. Artificial chemical stress has been produced by injecting an animal with the stress hormone.

- Stress can increase the triglyceride fraction of blood fat by 50 percent. (Triglycerides are the storage form of fat considered crucial in the development of heart disease.) Here is another stress/heart disease connection.

- People viewing sexually arousing films with others present, medical students who have just taken an oral exam and a group being interviewed for a job all have something in common: a rise in free fatty acids in their blood. Free fatty acids are organic acids that combine with glycerin (a sugar) to form fat. Even mild emotional stress produces an increase in free fatty acids in your blood. The researchers conclude that chronic anxiety probably leads to chronic elevation of fatty acids in the blood. This is why cholesterol levels go up when you are under stress.

- When test animals are isolated, which induces stress, the muscular tissue of their hearts has very low magnesium levels. This is one reason that loneliness actually causes physical impairment.

- When test animals are injected with the hormones secreted under stress, they are more likely to develop cancer. This is why it has been theorized that people under stress are more likely to be cancer victims.

- The effect of academic stress on immunity was measured in dental students by checking their salivary secretions for immunoglobulin, the protein which has antibody activity. The immunoglobulin secretion rate was significantly lower in high-stress than low-stress periods for the entire group.

- People undergoing a substantial number of life-change events show an increased incidence of allergic responses. Hospitalization is a life-change event.

- Experimental stress is associated with an increase in the number and severity of dental caries.

- The incidence of infectious mononucleosis among West Point cadets was highest among those in academic difficulty and whose parents had invested most in their success.

We believe that if your stress mechanisms are well-nourished, they will not break down. Nor should it be forgotten that the perception of stress may be altered by judicious relaxation, resignation and philosophy, because emotional stress is a personalized interpretation of external events. Again, repeated acute stressors result in chronic stress symptoms.

Your patient's stress stems not only from what actually

happened yesterday, but also what that patient anticipates will happen tomorrow.

The stress test

Here is a stress test that lists symptoms which may be an indicator of stress. The nurse may use this test for self-assessment, or as a discussion tool with patients.

Are you:

1 generally irritable, hyperexcited or depressed?
2 experiencing episodes of heart pounding?
3 experiencing a dry throat and mouth?
4 behaving impulsively, with aggression and emotional instability (emotion winning over logic)?
5 experiencing overpowering urges to cry or to run and hide?
6 unable to concentrate, "flighty" and generally disoriented?
7 accident prone?
8 having feelings of unreality, weakness or dizziness?
9 feeling fatigued and going through the day without "joie de vivre"?
10 having "floating anxiety," afraid without cause?
11 emotionally tense, alert and "keyed up"?
12 experiencing sexual difficulties, amenorrhea, impotence, premenstrual tension, or the "Casanova" complex, nymphomania?
13 trembling, with nervous tics?
14 easily startled by small sounds?
15 laughing with a nervous high pitch?

16 stuttering, or having other speech difficulties?

17 grinding the teeth—bruxism?

18 unable to sleep, a consequence of being "keyed up"?

19 having an increased tendency to move about or gesticulate without any apparent reason?

20 sweating excessively?

21 urinating frequently?

22 experiencing diarrhea, constipation, indigestion, queasiness in the stomach, or vomiting?

23 having no appetite, or an excessive one, showing itself in alterations of body weight—either excessive leanness or obesity?

24 experiencing pain in the neck or lower back?

25 having migraine headaches?

26 increasing smoking habits?

27 using additional prescribed medications, particularly tranquilizers or amphetamines?

28 addicted to alcohol or drugs?

29 experiencing nightmares?

30 experiencing neurotic behavior or even severe mental illness?

You cannot expect your patients to be completely free of stress. (We would worry about a hospitalized patient who did *not* experience stress.) The idea is to maximize the benefits of stress (such as motivation for behavior change) and to reduce its negative aspects.

Regardless of the ultimate manifestation of specific responses to stress, it all starts in your patient's brain; the hypothalamus defines an uncomfortable image, and relays this message to the networks, which in turn set up the barriers.

Table talk: stress

Is it possible to consume foods which supply an abundance of those nutrients that are wiped out by emotional stress? What are those nutrients? Studies show the following:

- Acetylcholine is formed from choline, which is mostly extracted from ingested foods. As indicated, people under stress need increased amounts of acetylcholine. Isn't it interesting that acetylcholine levels increase in depression and decrease in mania?

Choline-containing foods include egg yolks, organ meats, brewer's yeast, whole grains, soy beans, fish, legumes and lecithin.

- When under stress, large amounts of ascorbic acid are lost, particularly from the adrenal cortex. The intense breakdown induced by severe stress is also associated with loss of proteins, carbohydrates and fats. The protein is lost because ascorbic acid is necessary for the manufacture of some of the amino acids (the basic elements of protein). Constituents of protein are not properly formed when ascorbic acid supplies are diminished.

Vitamin C is utilized quickly and excreted easily. Within a few hours, half the supply is gone. If provisions were low to begin with, it may take up to twelve or thirteen hours to replenish, regardless of quantity ingested. And why should supplies be depleted? Dr. Irwin Stone, world-renowned ascorbic acid researcher, says:

> The human race has a genetic defect. We are missing an enzyme which is needed to produce ascorbic acid. A goat is

about the same size as an average human being, and is therefore a good animal for comparison. When a goat is relaxed (and quietly grazing on tin cans and long-playing records), it will produce about 13 grams of ascorbic acid per day. However, when stressed, the manufacture of ascorbic acid is increased to about one hundred or more grams. I believe that any human under any kind of stress will benefit greatly from increased intake of ascorbic acid.

Ascorbic acid foods include citrus fruit, rose hips, acerola cherries, alfalfa seeds, green vegetables, cantaloupe, strawberries, broccoli, tomatoes and green peppers.

• At least a dozen studies have shown that serotonin precursors improve mood disorders. (A precursor is a substance from which another substance is made.) Serotonin is a chemical messenger that transmits impulses between brain cells. Research has shown that serotonin levels are lower in brains of people who are depressed. So the question arises: do people become depressed because of low serotonin levels, or is serotonin lower in people who are depressed? In any case, if adequate quantities of amino acids are not available, the manufacture of serotonin is impaired. Tryptophan, a very important amino acid, is a significant precursor of serotonin; it is necessary for the manufacture of serotonin.

Foods containing tryptophan include nuts and seeds, organ meats, brown rice, carrots, beets, celery, endive, dandelion greens, fennel, snap beans, brussels sprouts, chives and alfalfa.

• Stress of any kind depletes the body of zinc. In some people, stress causes urine excretion of a substance called kryptopyrrole, which takes with it both zinc and vitamin B6.

Zinc-containing foods include sunflower seeds, seafood,

organ meats, mushrooms, brewer's yeast, soybeans, eggs and whole grains. Foods rich in vitamin B6 are yeast, whole grains, organ meats, egg yolks, legumes, green leafy vegetables, desiccated liver and muscle meats.

- The metabolic effects of chromium deficiency are greatly exaggerated in animals subjected to stress. One of these effects mimics that of insulin deficiency.

Chromium-containing foods are clams, whole grains and brewer's yeast.

- Is it any wonder that patients are so tired? Stress often causes the urinary excretion of acids which chelate (grab) iron and other metals, removing them from the body.

Foods containing iron are organ meats, egg yolks, fish, oysters, clams, whole grains, beans, green vegetables and desiccated liver.

- Again, the adrenal gland handles emotional stress via hormone regulation. Pantothenic acid supports this gland. When pantothenic acid-deficient diets are served to test subjects, they quickly become emotionally upset, irritable, quarrelsome, sullen, depressed and dizzy.

Foods containing pantothenic acid are organ meats, brewer's yeast, eggs, legumes, sweet potatoes, whole grains and salmon.

- Among the consequences of having too many free fatty acids in the blood (as a result of stress) is the reduction of magnesium. Magnesium is also lost when hormones are secreted during times of stress. These same hormones interfere with the cellular magnesium/calcium ratio. Magnesium protects the arterial lining from the mechanical stresses caused by sudden changes in blood pressure.

Magnesium-containing foods are vegetables, whole grains, raw dried beans and peas, seafood and nuts.

- Hormones secreted as a result of stress cause a decrease in the essential ratio of potassium to sodium both within and without the cell.

Your body does make heroic attempts to defend itself against the negative effects of stress. Adrenocorticotrophic hormone (ACTH), the adrenal hormone released under stress, is responsible for the release of substances which increase blood pressure needed to cope with stress. It accomplishes this mission by encouraging the retention of sodium and the excretion of potassium. This results in water retention, the consequence of which may be hypertension. Increased circulating blood fluid is one of the most dangerous aspects of hypertension.

Unprocessed foods contain more potassium than sodium—even those foods that are high in sodium. Food processing often reverses this ratio by decreasing potassium and adding salt. For example, a portion of fresh peas contains about one milligram of sodium and 380 milligrams of potassium. This ratio is beneficial to your cells. An equal portion of canned peas contains 230 milligrams of sodium and only 180 milligrams of potassium. This is a set-up for malfunction. Cells begin to scream out, "CANNOT COMPUTE," and if there is enough reason to protest, some cells see their final hour.

Foods high in potassium are lean meats, whole grains, vegetables, legumes, sunflower seeds and bananas.

How many, if any, foods on the patient's tray can replace nutrients lost to stress? Or is this another Catch-22 situation? Stress causes malnourishment, and *malnourishment causes stress.*

Calming nutrients

More than forty-five years ago vitamin E was described as "dampening the transmission of anxiety impulses from the thalamus (emotional brain) to the cortex (thinking brain)." Inositol, a factor of the vitamin B complex, has a quieting effect on the brain which, when displayed on an electroencephalograph, is curiously close to that of tranquilizers, *without the side effects*. Pantothenic acid, also a B-complex factor, helps the body tolerate stress better. Niacinamide, which acts upon the same cell receptors as do tranquilizers, quiets some individuals.

More information on the importance of niacin comes from a study conducted in Sweden. Volunteer subjects were placed under stress, and as expected, fatty acids, triglycerides, heart rate and blood pressure increased. A control group, exposed to the same stress, was given 3 grams of niacin. In this group, fatty acids and triglyceride levels were reduced. (Heart rate and blood pressure rose.)

It is interesting that our culture sees eggs as the culprit in the cholesterol discussion. The fact that stress increases cholesterol and triglyceride levels is rarely mentioned.

Other stress reducers

Exercise is a most important stress reducer because it has multiple benefits. It may be a challenge, however, to get inactive patients to move. For those who are reluctant or unable to move easily, you can encourage balloon blowing, or moving toes and fingers up and down, if that is all they can do. A rocker, if available, can serve for the very resistant. The action used for putting the rocker into motion stretches leg muscles and also stimulates circulation.

Other stress reducers may be flowers on a table (please find the time to water patients' flowers), relaxing music, natural lighting and a warm blanket. Sometimes the best way to determine the best means of reducing stress is simply to ask, "What can I do now to make you more comfortable?"

It is inadvisable to use the explicit term *stress* with a patient, because there are different interpretations of the word. You don't want to be involved in an intellectual discussion if you want to reduce stress. Naturally, stress reduction depends on many factors, and as always, you are the best judge of your nursing care, because you are guided by your instincts, knowledge and intuition.

Bibliography

Corsello, S. "Stress and Micronutrient Malabsorption." Presented at the First Forum of Nutritional Medicine, San Francisco, March 1983. Researched by Serafina Corsello and Betty Kamen.

Cox, T. *Stress* (Baltimore: University Park Press, 1978).

Kamen, B. and Kamen, S. *In Pursuit of Youth: Everyday Nutrition for Everyone Over 35* (New York: Dodd, Mead, 1984).

Jemmott, J. B. et al. "Academic Stress, Power Motivation, and Decrease in Secretion Rate of Salivary Secretory Immunoglobulin A." *Lancet* 1(1983):1400.

Selye, H. *The Stress of Life* (New York: McGraw-Hill Book Co., 1976).

Stroebel, C. *QR: The Quieting Reflex* (New York: G. P. Putnam's Sons, 1982).

Wurtman, R. J. "Nutrients That Modify Brain Function." *Scientific American* 246(1982):50.

8
POLITICS AND PATIENT COUNSELING

If I thought there was no hope in effecting change in the hospital diet, I would give up. I am not giving up.
                    LISA MORRARO, R.N.

Institutional cooking is a term that sounds as heavy or lifeless as the food it produces. Its negative connotation influences our perceptions about changing food quality—we can't help but feel that it is an almost hopeless situation.

Our comments are not about the institutions themselves. Institutions reflect the population they serve and the professionals who work in them. The American public retains a strong belief in the four food groups. Health professionals support that belief. Our government sanctions the use of irradiated foods, and there is a wide acceptance of canned, frozen and microwaved meals. Given these realities, what do we do? Immediate change in institutional food preparation is not our immediate concern. However, you should focus on *how you can make a difference for your patient right now.* Even in hospitals where food is catered, there is always room for negotiating. Concerned nurses could constitute an advisory committee to discuss diet procedures and report on what is working and what is not working in terms of nutrition.

What small modifications can you encourage? What suggestions can you offer the family? What can you tell patients to help them meet their nutritional needs or desires? How can you be assured that your patient will have something nutritious to eat—food that will contribute to health and healing?

We are operating on the premise that: 1. you are interested enough and convinced about the value of nutritional support for your patient; and 2. you feel powerful enough to know you can make a difference.

Nutrition and institutional cooking

Institutional cooking has a well-earned reputation for mediocrity at best, and not meeting basic requirements at worst. If you wonder if it's worth your while to get involved, consider that your attempt to have your patient better nourished is some compensation for the nonnourishing activities that are necessary in the hospital—some of which you are directly involved in and actively promote. (How many permits have you witnessed for procedures with side effects that are unknown to you?) Many of your patients' treatments, including medications and testing procedures, as well as being less mobile than usual, contribute negatively to their health. Nutrition can make a significant difference.

Another obvious issue is that nurses are hired to nurse, and nutrition is not generally regarded as an important part of that care—at least not when it comes to influencing what is on the meal tray. Yet nutritional status affects the outcome of care, and there is no one in a better position to assess that status than the nurse.

Nurses are expected to know and expound on the basic four food groups. When they deviate from these accepted guidelines, support from physicians and dieticians may erode. Nurses know there is a long time lapse between scientific discovery and acceptance of new facts. In the case of institutional cooking, we are up against very large business interests that are more concerned with cost control and efficiency than nutrition. If this sounds like a prophecy of doom, remember that you don't need to change more than a small part of that world for now.

Much of the information in this book may be new to many nurses, and perhaps even startling. Those who are responsible for institutional cooking may be equally uninformed, and would probably be resistant to ideas that challenge their basic assumptions (and may even threaten their jobs).

How nutritious is the food that is cooked in your institution? (We are not asking how nice or how hard-working the kitchen staff is.) How many fresh fruits and vegetables do you observe on the trays? How many are canned or frozen? Deep fried? Overcooked? How much raw food do you see? Are unrefined whole grains ever served? What about refined foods? What is the ratio between coffee and herbal teas? What are the choices?

Trust your own judgment and your ability to discriminate visually. We are not suggesting that institutions are serving foods that they think are nonnutritive or intentionally diminish a patient's health status. We are suggesting that you, as a health professional with a raised consciousness and an understanding of food and nutrition, assume responsibility to make some difference in your nusing care—within your own setting, institutional or not.

Personalizing nutrition

We know that it is not wise to attempt major changes in health behavior over a short time, especially when there are priorities apart from reevaluating nutritional status or needs. But as you plan your care in other areas, you can also plan nutritional care. Increasing fluids is a common practice in treating many illnesses. Let's set our sights higher.

Using your observational skills, you can determine some nutritional remedies that might help a particular patient. How often have you observed an impending ileus? Along with other nursing care you might give, you could add chamomile and peppermint tea to the diet. You could also reduce the nonnutritive, highly refined sugars and sodium solutions. Unrefined whole grains stimulate peristalsis. The teas and/or grains could be ordered from the kitchen or brought in by friends and family.

How do you respond to a productive cough? Would you like the secretion to be thinner and more easily expectorated?

Milk and cheese are mucus-producing foods. You could discourage the patient from drinking milk already on the tray with a brief explanation about its negative properties for this patient's illness.

When your patient wants a snack, what about a piece of fresh fruit instead of a sandwich? Food as a treatment for boredom or monotony is undesirable if it is nonnutritive.

How often do you see patients who are depressed, anxious, fatigued or lethargic? Illness and hospitalization may contribute or predispose to these attitudes. So can sugars and refined foods.

A physician was asked if he thought it would be a good idea to restrict milk consumption for patients who were obviously having difficulty with excess respiratory secretions. His response was that a number of his patients had told him that they chose to limit milk products in their diet because it resulted in less secretion. He added that he didn't think it worked in every case. Our thought was, how long would a drug be given if it had an adverse effect on *many*, but not *all* people? Those with respiratory difficulties already may be considered at risk for mucus-producing foods in their diet. (Nurses can influence how much or what foods are consumed from the tray. "Why don't you eat these foods first and see how you feel?")

You can create a rationale for deviations from institutional food. Ask patients how they feel after eating a particular meal. How much energy do they have? Do they feel good, and not just full? Do they feel too full and stuffed? Tired? Any headache? Any heart palpitation (a common symptom after consuming food to which one is sensitive)? Do they feel "comfortable" or irritable? Angry about being in the hospital or accepting? (Food and mood have been recognized as partners.) The patient's preference may have more power or influence for the physician than what you, the nurse, think is a good idea.

Encouraging patients to eat all of their nonnourishing food—whether they want it or not—may be counterproductive. "Finish what's on your plate" was an admonition that many of us heard as we grew up. "Listen to your body" is an admonition of choice. This is not to deny that some patients need encouragement to eat.

An assessment of the patient's preferences and experiences provide a data base for your activity. At that point you can determine whether the institution can modify what is on the tray, or whether you should focus on the family to see if it may provide for the patient directly.

Knowing the rules

Working within the realm of the institution requires knowing the rules. If there is a menu for patient selection, you have considerable power in helping the patient complete the menu. Getting the kitchen to comply with the patient's requests may be part of your work. Asking about alternate foods that could be added may be helpful. Citing that a patient has difficulty digesting or swallowing, or that a patient will only eat foods prepared in a particular way because of illness or preference, may garner some support from the kitchen staff.

If there is a supervisor who is responsible for special requests, be sure that person is contacted. Your concern is that your patient is provided with food that he or she will eat. Remember that for now your influence is limited. In the long run, however, you may contribute to improved food service.

Politics and Patient Counseling 155

Providing nontraditional nutritional care requires knowing the institution's rules. What are your facility's policies regarding food brought in to patients, and then perhaps stored? If there are limitations, how can exceptions be made? The classic case is that of immigrant patients who find American food distasteful and are reluctant to ask for special foods that might not even be available. For these patients it seems appropriate to allow food to be brought in. Needless to say, the physician's diet orders must be observed. If a low-salt or soft diet is the order of the day, this requirement should be heeded.

The next question is: if exceptions can be made for a foreign patient, why not for anyone else? If it is policy (and unless it is in writing, it may not be policy) to have approval before allowing food to be brought in, then discuss the issue with the person responsible. Mention that the patient feels that these foods are important for recovery. By noting the significance of food changes or preferences, you remove some of the emotional charge created with your decision to take on the task of food gatekeeper. Furthermore, when you emphasize that the patient is concerned about the type of food consumed, you are making a statement about how the diet directly relates to the patient's course of healing and recovery. You are reinforcing that patient's sense of autonomy and participation in his or her own care.

If there are no facilities for storing food brought in, inform the family or friends. Perhaps a thermos or small ice chest could be used. Containers of chemical ice (frozen at home) keep perishables under "refrigerated" conditions for many hours. If kept at room temperature, all containers should be sealed to discourage pests. (If housekeeping informs you about a problem because of stored food, pay attention.)

Specific suggestions for family take-ins

Broth is an excellent food and beverage when freshly prepared at home. You can suggest to family members that they use this or a similar recipe:

2 quarts water; ½ cup rice (or millet or barley); ½ cup each diced onion, green pepper, celery, carrot, sweet potato, zucchini, mushrooms; 2 tablespoons of tamari; dash of pepper; clove of garlic; oregano; thyme.

Bring water to boil. Add rice (or other grain). Reduce heat and cover. Cook on low for ½ hour. Add tamari and vegetables and seasonings. Barely simmer for 1 to 2 hours. Remove garlic clove before serving.

The vegetables and the seasonings could be varied. If the patient sips this broth throughout the day, valuable electrolytes will be replaced. If the patient feels well enough, the vegetables should be eaten in addition to sipping the broth. We would like to see this kind of broth made available on every hospital floor. Just think of the new aroma hospital corridors would take on! Until the time that "The Broth" becomes standard prescription, the members of any family or any kind neighbor or friend could easily prepare this elixir.

Another valuable mix is a fresh preparation of vegetable juices, preferably a blend of carrot, celery, peppers and green leaves. This is more difficult to come by because it requires a juicerator and time. If there is a health store in the vicinity that sells mixed vegetable juices prepared as ordered, encourage the family to take advantage of this luxury. (Although less costly than most medicine, it's more expensive than apple juice. Remind everyone that food that doesn't nourish you is expensive.) Either of these special foods could be eaten as substitutes or additions to the institution's food.

A sacred cow in the hospital setting is fruit juice. Most nurses will offer these refined, sugary beverages to the patient with a firm belief that they have some vitamins and minerals. The bad news is that these beverages, though tasty and convenient, are just another form of concentrated simple carbohydrates, with the minimal retention of nutrients of junk food. You may not remove these from a patient's diet, but you may match the glasses of fruit drink with a glass of water. "Force fluids" does not mean to be indiscriminate with liquids.

Sprouts are another excellent food, if available. The sprouted seed is one of the most nutritious foods. Each seed contains an embryo which is a miniature of what the plant will be. Sprouts are harvested at the point where the seed is manufacturing all those life-giving nutrients. Many of the sprout proteins are predigested—they are converted to amino acids during the sprouting process. The starches are also converted to simple sugars requiring little digestive breakdown, so they enter the bloodstream rapidly and are classed as a quick-energy food.

Sprouts also contain enzymes, and have been shown to be hormone stimulators. They are nutrient-dense foods. Doesn't this sound like ideal fare for patients on the mend? Several types of sprouts are available in grocery or health food stores. Many varieties can be home-grown.

If your institution requires written orders for foods brought in (which is not likely), then ask for them or ask the patients or a family member to express their needs. An outspoken family member or friend can be the patient's best ally in communicating with the physician or dietician.

Why should a patient have to wait to get out of a health-care institution before engaging in such basic health-giving therapy as eating nourishing foods?

Institutions and interactions

The politics that immediately affect the nurse are those involving interactions with other nursing staff, physicians and dieticians. Why should the nurse want to actively participate in any more politics than necessary? Because the stakes are high, and much is to be gained for the patient. But perhaps you have to answer that question for yourself.

Dealing with an institution may seem easy in comparison to dealing one-to-one with the professionals who share responsibility with patients under your care.

The physician's formal training offers the same limited knowledge of nutrition that some nursing programs offer. Information received subsequently often comes from major food producers who of course reinforce the notion of the four food groups as they promote processed foods. The same is true of the dieticians' source of information. This is not a judgment as to who is right or wrong; it is a statement of fact. (We would rather focus on what works.)

It may not be wise to expect these groups to be your allies as you develop and emphasize your own beliefs about nutritious foods. The beneficial effect of the many dietary changes we suggest may not be detected immediately. But these facts should not deter your involvement.

You may be asked for references from professionals. When you respond with, "The information is in the literature," you are likely to be asked, "Where?" Use references from this book for starters. (Keep copies of some pages with you at work.)

On more than one occasion we have been asked to deliver data for a physician's perusal. Care must be taken not to slip into the role of librarian or research assistant. If there is a medical librarian available, interested parties can get the information without your help. How much time you devote to educating other RNs or MDs depends on the relationship you have with them, and what the expected effect may be on the patient.

The role of the physician

In our experience, physicians are often amenable to requests to add "peppermint and chamomile tea" to the diet order. One hospital food service has called out for smoked salmon, but is mystified about how to get millet. Asking the physician for special diet orders may be required, even if the request is for a faster advancement of diet than anticipated by the doctor. With the physician's permission, you can notify the kitchen and, using his or her name, tell them how important the request is to the MD.

Is there research that supports the diet orders for postcesarean women? The requests range from NPO to regular diets. If there were hard data for physicians, how could the orders vary so dramatically? Some postoperative patients must pass flatus before solid food is given. Hot chamomile and/or peppermint teas facilitate peristalsis, as does ambulation. After the first passing of flatus, the physician could be notified *per patient request*, so that the diet could be advanced, if this means that a patient could have the advanced diet a full day sooner. The point is that diet orders are often made arbitrarily. These orders could be changed.

Physicians want their patients to be comfortable and satisfied, and the nurse is in an excellent position to promote this. If your efforts to improve your patient's nutritional status mean a healthier patient, and you carry out the required effort in a pleasant, professional manner, there should be no concern. And sometimes the physician will say—even before the nurse does—that the important thing is to do what works. Easy for them to say, you might respond, because they are not bound by as many orders as you, the nurse. Nor do they need to keep asking for permission to do what is obviously called for.

Dieticians have been schooled in the same tradition as physicians. And again, we are not saying this is wrong. But we do question whether traditional and familiar positions should be maintained and defended in light of current research. Nursing is not exactly progressive in its approach to nutrition, but the nurse's territory appears to be more "open" to a holistic approach.

To be or not to be involved

Whether you want to participate actively in your patient's nutritional status is a question only you can answer. You have to determine whether you feel it is in your patient's best interest at the time. You must also consider the many obstacles you will face, including your own energy expenditure. Anyone involved in nursing today, either actively or inactively, knows that the shrinking health dollar and emphasis on profit affect all levels of care. Resources for nursing care are not what they used to be. Compounded with the new technology for treatment, including new and more powerful drugs, are the advances in food technology, placing all of us at greater risk.

Because eating is so personal, your interest in the patient's diet is an expression of concern and warmth—an outstretched hand. More than that, you are offering assurance that the patient has an internal healing system, one that can respond favorably if properly nourished. Inner healing may be the most important reason to be involved in more nutritious eating.

We want to speak to the "shoulds" that are inherent in discussions such as these. There is no reason you "should" chase down some herbal tea or fresh fruit or nurturing broth for a patient. Do that if you have the time and interest. Nursing is already replete with guilt-producing elements, and now that you have more knowledge about nutrition, you can feel good about seeking information. If situations appear to be impossible to deal with, you should know when to move on. That doesn't mean that you have failed in your attempt to improve patient care. It does mean you have made a choice about where to put your energy. Knowing the limits of a situation is important in any discussion.

When you make the choice to share nutrition education with your patient, be aboveboard. We often suggest that patients discuss nutrition with their physicians. This imparts a strong message to the patient, by indicating that no covert activity is going on, and that the physician is interested in the patient's nutrition. It tells the patient that the doctor supports the patient's own ability to mobilize the body to turn back disease. Now the patient has the choice of pursuing the suggestions or not.

Patients need to be advised that there are many controversies concerning diet (as if that is news to anyone), and that it is the patient who must ultimately choose what he or she is consuming. We can hardly count the times new mothers expressed surprise that they could choose whether to give their newborns sugar water or plain water. "Why didn't anyone tell me I had a choice?" is the most frequent response. (We do not advocate routine water supplementation for breast-fed infants.)

The extent of your commitment to nutrition reeducation may vary from the suggested use of herbal teas to encouraging the use of vegetarian cookbooks to expand at-home culinary repertoire. A certain amount of risk-taking activity is called for in any matter of change. Just because territory and routine are threatened, avoidance behavior is not the answer. Nurses have certainly traversed more difficult arenas than this, and with less at stake.

The hospital or health care setting is an ideal place in which to introduce concepts that may alter a person's health care status. Some have questioned whether the patient should be burdened, and we respond by pointing out that this may be the best time for intervention. We do not suggest a major restructuring of food beliefs, but applicable concepts can be introduced at this time. We are dealing with a motivated population, even if its focus is on care with a more immediate perceived benefit.

Nurses could choose to avoid the issue, letting the patient deal with food changes later. There is no "later" for most of our patients, no time that will be as good as the present. Attention to rest and to mobilization and activity are all "now" issues, as well as the tests, treatments and medications. Why should food be relegated to *later*, when the need is most dramatic *now*, and in fact intervention can make a difference in the course of recovery?

Nursing is both science and art. A patient's treatment is not complete if it is limited to medical diagnosis and the administration of medicines, or to nursing diagnoses that avoid nutrition. The patient's own resources and capacities should be involved, and what better way to do this than to teach how to make good food choices? Giving medicine and performing some nursing functions are science. Teaching is an art.

"Are you a health nut?" is a question you should not be surprised to hear once you start this process. You can also expect that people will watch to see if you eat sweets, to determine whether you practice what you preach. When we are asked if we are "health nuts," we may respond, "I don't know what you mean. What is a health nut?"

The human healing system has been honed by three million years of evolution and about fifty years of invasive intervention. The hospital can do a better job of providing a setting for human life and healing than it is doing now.

We know we are asking for a reassessment of your own attitudes toward nutrition. We do not underestimate the challenge. We also know that nurses constitute the largest group of health professionals in the country. You have tremendous influence.

To paraphrase a common saying, nutrition reeducation, support and monitoring are jobs that someone has to do, and no professional is better suited or situated than the nurse.

Bibliography

Beeber, L. S. and Schmitt, M. H. "Cohesiveness in Groups: A Concept in Search of a Definition." *ANS* 8(1986):1.

Connor, S. L.; Gustafson, J. M.; and Vaughan, S. R. "Promoting Dietary Change." *Journal of the American Dietetic Association* 85 (1985): 345.

Editorial. "Are They Being Served?" *Lancet* 1(1985):1491.

Jones, M. G.; Bonner, J. L.; and Stitt, K. R. "Nutrition Support Service: Role of the Clinical Dietician." *Journal of the American Dietetic Association* 86(1986):68.

Morris, D. H. and Lubin, A. H. "A Review of the Symposium 'Diet and Behavior: A Multidisciplinary Evaluation.'" *Association of Medical Professionals* 77(1985):256.

9

LIVING WHAT YOU ARE TEACHING

The germ is nothing. The terrain is everything.

LOUIS PASTEUR

We all live in interaction with our entire environment. It is not enough that the air we breathe, the water we drink and the food we eat all contain untold billions of microorganisms, viruses, pollutants, toxins and as yet unidentified substances. For you, the nurse, there is above-average exposure.

Can you protect yourself from the occupational hazards of the hospital? We have discussed the need for greater emphasis on nutrition in nursing care. What about *your* nutrition?

The nurse at risk

Articles defining measures to prevent infection among nurses occupy a lot of space in medical journals. The approach to infection control is often "bugs and drugs" (which organisms are controlled by which drugs), or "rules, routines and rituals" (if we follow the rules, and routinely wash or spray with this or that, we will be infection-free). But the very substances used as antiseptics may be toxic!

Anticancer agents represent a class of occupational carcinogens. The urine of nurses working in oncology wards has been shown to be more mutagenic than that of nurses in other units. Absorption of chemotherapy drugs mixed before administration to patients takes place either through the skin or through inhalation.

Two recent studies involving hospital personnel point to increased risks of pregnancy disorders. One of the studies showed an excess of spontaneous abortions, and the other malformations in children of women who worked with anticancer agents. Statistics show a greater percentage of infertility among nurses than in the general population.

What emerges is the fact that nurses are at high risk. It would seem that it should be incumbent that nursing instructors teach their students that *if body mechanisms are well nourished, they will not break down as easily as those that are malnourished.*

Isn't it just plain common sense that people who are better nourished have more resistance to disease? We have had our "double blind" studies for centuries—observations which prove this fact again and again, and yet again. Shouldn't common sense dictate that we place more credibility in therapies that have been tried and true and effective for generations, rather than on those which have been used for a shorter time? The more advertising a treatment has had from its manufacturers, the more popular it becomes. No one pays to advertise the benefits of breast feeding or parsley. Common sense should dictate at least some skepticism with so much that is so new.

The problems of personal change

Of course we can intellectualize about good eating habits. We all agree that eating a variety of healthful foods is in everyone's best health interest. Altering lifelong habits, however, is another matter. There's no magic bullet, no solution-in-a-pill. An ancient Chinese proverb says, "Person would sooner give up spouse than give up customary dietary."

Many have given nutrition the old college try and failed. Our friend Toby is an example. When she had witnessed too many deaths in the course of a few day's duty, she went home one night and emptied her kitchen of all nonnutritious bread. Second day: she threw out everything containing large amounts of processed sugar. Third day: she did away with sweet boxed breakfast cereals. Fourth day: her family got rid of *her*. The Tobys of the world say, "See, I tried it. It didn't work. What do I do now?"

Those who study the foodways of the late twentieth century usually discover more than they set out to find. And most of it is disturbing. Then they try to get friends and family to adopt concepts to improve life quality. They learn quickly how difficult it is to get others to overcome bad eating habits. (We are not discussing hospitalized patients whose motivations and immediate needs are very different from those of the general population.)

We all suffer thinly disguised self-deceptions (even the very same nutrition educators); we compromise and bargain so we may have our goodies. Knowing the rules does not exclude us from being hooked on *something*. Almost everyone manipulates to get a fix of coffee, sweets, booze or cheesecake (that's ours).

Although scientists claim to know the chemical assay of an orange, they have yet to create an orange in the laboratory. We know some of the complexities of nourishment. But we do not know nearly enough to intercept nature, and yet we produce cheese that isn't cheese (processed cheese food), raisins that aren't raisins (made from modified starch and sugar) and other synthetic foods that are nonfoods (ersatz butter, eggs, and so forth). Perhaps we will be able to accept the chemists' capability to nourish us with replacement food products when they can create an orange containing seeds which, if planted, will grow into an orange tree that produces more oranges.

So here we are with problems: 1. difficulty in change (it is not easy to intercept the warm shelter of habit; young children especially view change as betrayal); 2. foods that are adulterated; and 3. foods that are not real. Yet it has been demonstrated again and again that optimal health can only be achieved with optimal nourishment, the kind of food that is primal—food that has not been mushed, mashed and mangled. And yet to succeed in this business of health improvement, we cannot be rigid and unbending, nor can we alter things overnight.

Steps of change

To help temper the transition from Standard American Diet (note the acronym—it's SAD) to fare that is both healthful and welcome, we have developed a series of "steps of change." In addition to benefits for both you and your family, we believe you will be a much more effective care-giver after you have personally experienced the agonies and the ecstasies involved in the process of changing your own eating lifestyle.

CHANGE #1: GIVE BEFORE YOU TAKE AWAY

The first step for the kitchen in transition is to avoid resistance by adding instead of taking away. The master stroke is to remove nothing, but to lay out healthful snacks—raw vegetable strips in tiny attractive places; green peas still adhering to their protective pods for the kids to take apart, or for you to nibble while watching TV; sections of fruit on toothpicks; nuts and seeds in the shell to break open as evening snacks—treats that boast nutrition scattered around the house. Be sure to use products that have not gone into wilt or decline. The appeal of these snacks is not their vitamin, mineral or enzyme content, but rather their visual "invitingness" and the pleasure-giving quality of chewy and crackly foods. And remember that everyone is more comfortable with what is familiar. It's harder to urge new, unfamiliar foods on a reluctant family, or even on yourself. These same snacks can be packaged and taken to work.

We learn from vestiges of very early civilizations that food was an intrinsic part of culture. The importance of a favorable experience with food was considered equal to enjoyment derived from any other intellectual or esthetic happening. Therefore, the serving of food was an art form. Color, shape, harmony, texture, combination and even aroma were all vitally important. If the term "holistic" had been popular in the long ago, it would have been stated that it was culturally inherent for food to fit the holistic picture. The appearance of food was not divorced from its nutrition—the art of dispensing a meal was as important as the biochemistry of its nourishment. (At a time, for example, when the breakdown products of protein, the amino acids, were unknown, the combining of foods to produce complete protein was common practice.)

Reccntly it has been demonstrated that when we chew foods that are appetizing, we actually cause a greater increase in salivary flow than we produce when chewing less exciting foods.

Here are a few specific ideas for Steps of Change #1:

FIBER FEASTS

Season yogurt (for calcium and good-guy bacteria) with hulled sesame seeds (for health-giving nutrients of seeds in general, and the amino acid methionine in particular). Embellish the dip with tofu (for more calcium, protein, B vitamins and ease of digestion) and/or mashed avocado (for polyunsaturated fatty acids). Place in a small pretty dish and surround with strips of bright-colored, crisp cucumbers, zucchini, sweet red peppers, mushrooms and carrots (for fiber and minerals).

Vary the dip. Prepare *Tofu Mock Cottage Cheese.* ½ pound soft tofu; ¼ cup fresh parsley, finely chopped (for vitamin A, C, and iron); ¼ cup fresh scallions, minced (for potassium); ¼ cup sugar-free, additive-free mayonnaise (for polyunsaturated fatty acids); ½ teaspoon minced garlic (for antibiotic properties); 1 tablespoon cider vinegar (to help balance your pH). Let tofu drain in colander while cutting vegetables. Mash tofu into cottage-cheese texture. Combine all other ingredients with tofu; blend until creamy. Serve chilled. (Place bowl over slightly larger bowl of ice cubes.)

SWEET-TOOTH SATISFIERS

Mini-Marvels. 3 fertile eggs, well beaten (for first-rate protein—including rare sulfur amino acids); 1 cup freshly cracked and chopped walnuts (for more polyunsaturated fats); 8 ounces presoaked chopped dates or untreated raisins (mostly for the love affair we have with sweetness). Mix everything together. Spoon into greased and floured *tiny* muffin tins. Bake at 350°, 20 minutes. Makes 24 small taste treats. Note: you must use mini-tins. (Although a mini-marvel may not offer the exquisite delight of chocolate mousse, it's not bad. And it's a boon for the wheat-sensitive.)

Almond Crunch Chewies. ⅓ cup raw butter (for vitamin A); ¼ cup unfiltered raw honey (for some minerals and lots of flavor); ¾ cup slivered almonds (for vitamin B6). Melt butter in skillet; stir honey into butter. Add almonds. Cook at medium temperature. Stir while cooking. Takes about 6 to 8 minutes for mixture to turn golden-brown. Spread in prepared pan while mixture is still hot. Use oiled or buttered sharp knife to cut into squares while hot. After cooling, place in refrigerator in covered container.

Sweet Potato Snack. When you prepare your dinner, throw a sweet potato or two into the oven. Let this vitamin A-, C- and mineral-packed goody sit around after cooking, and hold in abeyance until the family is looking for a tasty, filling, tempting snack later on. Serve this golden, sweet feast in thick slices on toothpicks. (Underbake slightly so that the potato is still firm, not soft. Overcooked potatoes have the same deleterious effect on blood sugar as sweet desserts.) If your family is not too salt/sweet-saturated, they may even look for seconds.

This first stage of the kitchen in transition should help to provide some of the frequently missed nutrition links in the day's diet. But remember—these suggestions should be *in addition to*, not *in place of* the usual. Substitutions at the outset create feelings of deprivation. Let's approach that step cautiously.

CHANGE #2: NO-SALT INSURANCE

Now we get to the nitty-gritty. We're going to "shake it out." Step #2 is to eliminate the salt shaker.
A full page ad in *FDA Consumer*, October 1985, offers a free poster to encourage people to curtail the use of salt. The FDA wants everyone to know that sodium is in almost every food you eat, but that if you get too much of it, high blood pressure and other diseases may develop.
Is it possible to remove a favorite food enhancer and not have you or family members feel deprived? We say yes—once you learn to use the range of herbs, spices and other flavor contributors that add pungency and perhaps an even more exciting personality to everyday foods.
Most American kitchens already contain a supply of herbs. Sadly, they are almost always stored near the stove where they rest in an atmosphere too warm for nutrient retention. But no matter—they are rarely used: chances are they are as old as the racks which support them.
For those to whom *haute cuisine* means adding a dash of pepper after sprinkling an abundance of salt, it may be expe-

dient to purchase prepared herb mixes which clearly designate their destiny. For example, you can buy an Oriental combo for stir-fry; Italian blend for garlic bread; French mix for casseroles and soups; and an all-purpose merge for all purposes. Or, if you are more adventurous, you can lay in a supply of oregano, parsley, rosemary, basil, capsicum, chili powder, garlic, thyme, tarragon, sage, a bay leaf or two and so on. Either way, please store the condiments in a cool place, and discard—or use in your bath—if not consumed in four months. (For economy, share your purchases with a friend or neighbor.)

The next step is to transform the simplest fare into a gastronomic treat so that the salt shaker won't be missed. For the diehards who salt before they taste, the following herbs have a salty flavor: summer savory, lovage and celery. These herbs are easiest to use if dried or powdered. Or, while in transition, you could replace the contents of the salt shaker with this composite: one tablespoon of ground coarse salt (coarse salt has more flavor than the overprocessed free-flowing variety, so you use less), ¼ tablespoon each of ground black peppercorns, ground coriander seeds, ground bay leaves and dried basil. Slowly reduce the salt content and increase other condiments. (See also *Tasty Salt Substitute* in the recipe section below.)

HERB-TO-TASTE

Start your cooking changeover with an herb omelet for Sunday breakfast—an omelet so flavorful and aromatic that no one will think of picking up the salt shaker (see recipe below). Try cinnamon on oatmeal or other cereals to replace salt. Melted sweet butter with oregano can be served over fish. There are no rigid rules, but here's a beginner's herb guide:

Food	Herbs to use
Butter spreads	caraway, chives, garlic, parsley, tarragon
Eggs	basil, coriander, cress, dill, parsley, tarragon, thyme
Fish	basil, chives, dill, fennel, parsley, tarragon, sesame seeds
Meats	basil, dill, marjoram, mint, oregano, rosemary, sage, thyme
Poultry	basil, dill, lemon balm, lovage, rosemary, sage, tarragon, thyme
Salad and salad dressings	basil, chives, cress, dill, garlic, marjoram, oregano, parsley, savory, tarragon
Soups	basil, bay leaf, chives, dill, oregano, parsley, tarragon; capsicum, cumin, curry powder for "hot" soup.

VEGETABLES

Squash, turnips	basil
Onions	bay leaf or saffron
Cabbage, carrots	dill
Peas, spinach	marjoram
Mushrooms	oregano
Green beans	rosemary
Beans	sage
Lentils, lima beans	savory
Asparagus, celery	tarragon
Beets	thyme

Most herbs should be added in moderation during the last stages of cooking. If cooked too long, they may give a bitter taste to foods.

Mild herbs are sage, rosemary, savory, chervil, chives and parsley, and those with stronger flavors include oregano, basil, dill, thyme, marjoram, bay, mint and tarragon. Fresh herbs are preferable when available. Rule of thumb is to use twice the amount of fresh herbs as dried. Dried herbs have a stronger, more concentrated flavor.

A "bouquet garni" can be added to soups or stews. Use any three or more of the following (tied together if you have fresh herbs; placed in a little sac if chopped or ground): bay leaf, thyme, chervil, basil, marjoram and savory. Discard after cooking. Whether you use a sprig or a bundle of herbs depends on your family's taste. Again, there are no rules.

A few more quick herb hints to try: bruised garlic clove and twist of orange peel for meat while cooking; chopped chervil leaves for cream soups; dill for consommé or sliced tomatoes; chives and/or chervil for baked potatoes; mint for potatoes or peas; thyme for turkey; sage for cheese dips; basil over baked apples; savory for deviled eggs; chives to add oniony flavor to anything.

CAVEAT EMPTOR

There are a wide variety of processes available for producing dried or concentrated foods. Any single process involves a range of conditions which affect the nutrient retention of the final product. Manufacturers producing supplies for natural food stores are usually more aware of methods which retain more nutrients, and are more apt to limit additives.

RECIPES

Tasty Salt Substitute. Blend or grind 1 teaspoon each of garlic flakes, cumin seed, black peppercorns, brewer's yeast flakes. Blend 1 teaspoon each of parlsey flakes, onion flakes, bell pepper flakes, celery seed, kelp powder. Add to first mixture.

This recipe can be modified by adding small quantities of the following: oregano, toasted sesame seeds, toasted squash or pumpkin seeds, caraway seeds or dried mushrooms.

176 Nutrition in Nursing: The New Approach

Tarragon Vinegar Salad Dressing. Combine ¼ teaspoon pepper; ¼ teaspoon dry mustard; 1 teaspoon Dijon mustard; 3 tablespoons tarragon vinegar; 8 tablespoons oil; 1 raw egg; 1 finely chopped garlic clove. Mix thoroughly.

TNT Salad—Tomato-and-Thyme. Heap romaine in salad bowl; add garlicked squares of bread, two sliced tomatoes, and several paper-thin slices of onion separated into rings. Add 1 tablespoon tarragon. Dress with olive oil, pepper and vinegar.

Sauce For Fish. 2 tablespoons butter; 1 green onion; ½ clove garlic; 1 tablespoon minced parsley; ¼ teaspoon thyme; ¼ teaspoon marjoram; ½ teaspoon sage. Melt butter, mince in onion and garlic. Cook gently 5 minutes. Add parsley and other herbs. Stir, cook 5 minutes more. Mix well. Pour over fish before serving.

Omelet With Fine Herbs. Use 8-inch frying pan. 4 eggs; dash of black pepper; 1 teaspoon chopped parsley; ½ teaspoon chopped chives; 2 tablespoons butter. Beat eggs lightly. Add pepper. Add herbs and mix slightly. Melt butter in pan until it covers bottom. Roll pan so butter coats sides. When butter is bubbling briskly, but still uncolored, pour in eggs. As soon as edges are set, run spatula under its center so all uncooked portions run underneath cooked part. Do this from time to time. When omelet is café-au-lait underneath, and creamy on top, fold over in middle and coax off pan onto hot platter. Serve at once. (Like time and tide, omelets wait for no one!)

CHANGE #3: GAIN WITH GRAINS—AND WE DON'T MEAN POUNDS

Buckwheat (or kasha) graces every Russian table. The Chinese eat a lot of rice; Mexicans, corn. Europeans love rye.

Oats and Irish have been dubbed synonyms. In Africa, millet is a staple. These patterns of grain eating developed independently in all parts of the world. Recent high-tech research offers an understanding of why the patterns work so well, and why they endure. Today, more people rely on grains for energy than any other type of food. Americans, however, eat virtually no whole grains—even though we are one of the world's largest grain producers. The addition of whole grains is Step #3 on the food-change continuum.

WHY GRAINS AND WHICH GRAINS

Low cost, easy storage and a bundle of nutrients (fiber, iron, niacin, and thiamin) not found in meat or dairy products are just a few reasons why whole grains deserve more space on the American table. Here's a short list of grains which could give you a boost or two on the stay-healthy scale.

Wheat. The whole wheatberry is rich in vitamins B1 and E, protein, an array of minerals and natural fiber. Milled wheat is devoid of its germ or embryo and fiber coat, and it emerges with distorted protein structures. Even when enriched, only some of the stripped nutrients are returned, and then in synthetic form. Those who are sensitive to processed wheat products often find they can tolerate whole wheat, the unmilled variety.

Oats. Unlike wheat, the germ and the bran of the oat remain intact, even when commercially processed. Oats, however packaged, are always a whole grain. Oats are high in protein and fiber.

Buckwheat. Our country grew up on buckwheat pancakes. Let's make it a favorite again. Kasha is rich in iron and B vitamins, plus the amino acid lysine. The quality of buckwheat can be improved further if combined with sesame flour, which is high in methionine. Lysine and methionine are two amino acids in short supply in most plant foods. (Amino acids are the building blocks of protein.)

Millet. Millet is a grain eaten by millions of people in Asia and Africa daily—perhaps because it is one of the most nutritious of all grains. More nearly a complete protein than any other grain, it is also high in minerals, easily digested, incredibly adaptable, and has a bland, slightly nutty flavor.

Rice. The only disadvantage of whole brown rice when compared with white rice is cooking time; brown rice takes a bit longer, a small price to pay for B vitamins, fiber and quality protein. Because commercial rice is often heavily sprayed, this is one product that should be purchased in a natural-food store.

RECIPES

It is time to cut down on the consumption of grains in their least nutritious form—as commercial breads and cereals, pasta and pastries and overprocessed snacks. There are pleasant surprises in store when you move whole grains back into the arena of prime staples. They can be prepared with simplicity—cooked with some liquid and served as a porridge. (Cinnamon and sliced banana added to oatmeal can be good cheer on a cold winter morning.) Or whole grains can be elevated to a cuisine that rivals the most artful of edibles. (Oriental brown rice, described below, has the promise of becoming your new house specialty.)

Beware quick, instant or minute preparations. At the very least they are more processed (that's what makes them cook fast), and at worst they may have undesirable additives (again, to speed up the cooking).

Easy Millet. 1 cup water; ½ cup millet; cayenne pepper; sesame seeds. Boil water. Add millet. Lower heat and cook, covered, 15 to 20 minutes, or until all water is absorbed. Add dash of pepper and handful of sesame seeds. Optional: crushed garlic; small bits of avocado. Serves two or three.

Oriental Brown Rice. 4 tablespoons sesame oil; 1 cup brown rice; 2 cups water; 1 cup mushrooms; 1 cup bean sprouts; 1 cup chopped celery; 1 cup chopped red or green peppers; 4 cloves mashed garlic; 2 eggs; 1 cup green peas; 3 tablespoons tamari. Place 1 tablespoon oil in skillet; heat. Add rice slowly. (Coating rice with oil prevents sticking.) Pour water into another pot; boil. Add oil-coated rice slowly; cover. Reduce heat; set timer for 30 minutes. Add remainder of oil. Stir-fry mushrooms; set aside. Stir-fry rest of ingredients except for eggs, peas and tamari. Add tamari. Add rice; stir. Lightly scramble 2 eggs; toss into mixture. Add raw peas. *Optional*: Add 1 or 2 cups diced chicken or turkey. Serves two for main course, four or five for side dish.

Buckwheat Pancakes. 2 eggs; 2½ cups buttermilk; 2 tablespoons butter; 1 tablespoon honey; ½ cup whole wheat flour; 1½ cups buckwheat flour; 1½ teaspoons aluminum-free baking powder. Combine eggs and buttermilk. Add butter, then honey, and beat thoroughly. In separate container, stir together flours and baking powder, pressing out lumps. Add liquid ingredients, stirring only until blended. Add water if too thick, flour if too thin. Drop batter on slightly greased hot griddle. Cook until just a bit dry on top (bubbles will form); turn and cook on other side. Serve hot. Serves two.

Cheese Oat Cakes. 1 cup oats (or oat flakes); ½ cup oat flour; ½ cup sesame flour; ¼ cup softened butter; 1 cup sharp cheddar cheese, grated; ½ cup warm water. Stir together oatmeal and flour. Cut in butter with fork; stir in cheese. Add water and mix, kneading when dough is too stiff to stir. Separate dough into thirds, roll into circles, ¼-inch thick. Cut circles into wedges; bake on lightly greased baking sheet for 20 minutes at 400°.

Sweet Wheatberry Snack. Soak 2 tablespoons wheatberries in water overnight. Drain in morning. (Use drained water on your plants.) Spread wheatberries on platter. Leave on kitchen counter. Rinse and drain every morning and evening until sprouts are a bit longer than the berries—about two or three days. Add to salads or soups, or nibble as is. (The longer wheatberries sprout, the sweeter they become.) The germ (commonly known as wheat germ) plus the outer coating (referred to as bran) are left intact—an offering of vitamin E and fiber in a whole form.

Homemade Granola. 3 cups rolled oats; 1 cup whole wheat flour or sprouted wheatberries; ½ cup hulled sesame seeds; ½ cup walnuts; ½ cup sunflower seeds; ½ cup shredded coconut; ¼ cup oil; ⅛ cup honey. Preheat oven to 225°. Distribute mixture thinly on cookie sheet. Place in oven for 1 hour until lightly browned. Options: Eliminate honey. Add raisins, chopped dates, chopped apricots, dried apples, chopped prunes. (Options are added after granola has baked.) Store in tightly covered canister in cool place, or refrigerate.

Vegetarian Meatloaf. 1 cup sesame seeds; 2 cups cooked brown rice; 1 cup cooked millet; 1 cup cooked bulgur wheat; 1 cup cooked barley; 1½ cups ground unsalted raw peanuts; ½ cup ground almonds; 1½ cups sesame tahini; 4 tablespoons minced parsley; 2 teaspoons thyme; 2 tablespoons chopped chives; 2 minced carrots; 2 stalks of minced celery; 2 cups chopped mushrooms (small pieces); 4 teaspoons sesame oil; tamari to taste.

Heat oil in fry pan. Add minced vegetables and stir briefly. Add seasoning and tamari. Set aside in mixing bowl. Mix grain with nuts and seeds. Add tahini, blending well. The tahini acts as a natural binder and nutritonal booster. Now add vegetables to this. Lightly oil a glass pyrex dish and press mix into it. Preheat oven to 350° and bake 30 minutes. Serves eight.

CHANGE #4: ELIMINATE SIMPLE SUGAR TO AVOID COMPLEX DISEASE

Parting company with refined sugar in our culture is easier said than done. No one really understands why we have such a love affair with sweets. But eliminating refined sugar is essential if we are to progress on the health continuum.

Some people are secret sugarholics, hiding candy bars in the chandelier, tucking Twinkies under socks in the closet or filling official-looking attaché cases with Godiva chocolates. Others eat ice cream out in the open and keep jellybeans in plain sight on their desks. Either way, we expose ourselves to risk.

SUGAR ADDICTION

It is undisputed that heroin is not a natural ingredient of the daily diet. People become conditioned to the "high" of this physiologically addictive substance. After a while, a vicious cycle develops; in order to feel better, heroin must be reintroduced into the body. Everyone recognizes that this is heroin addiction. But people respond in a similar fashion to other addictive substances—coffee, cigarettes and *refined sugar.* If you abstain from any of these abruptly, you have withdrawal symptoms. Perhaps a headache. Possibly extreme fatigue. The symptoms of withdrawal can be worse than the symptoms caused by the intake of the addicting ingredient. The difference is that the withdrawal symptoms are temporary.

Refined sugar is a man-made substance introduced to us as a food since childhood. Many people no longer have enough internal equilibrium for the pancreas, liver and other glands to orchestrate the metabolizing of refined sugar. This is what leads to the conditioning that takes place exactly like any addictive drug response—the kind you see in alcohol and drug rehabilitation wards.

SWEET-TALK EDUCATION

So we have a double-edged sword. Not only do we feel deprived when the food we love is banished, but we also suffer very real physical discomfort. A partial solution is education. Every member of the family should understand why refined sugar is such a rascal. Everyone should know that the more processed a food is, the less nutrient value it has. *Refined sugar is just about the most processed food there is*; 90 percent of the original sugar cane or sugar beet is removed at the manufacturer's plant. Not one action of refined sugar can be considered beneficial. And far too many actions of sugar are disastrous. To cite but a few:

- A study reported in *Metabolism* demonstrated that feeding sucrose to those prone to hypertension raises blood pressure.
- Maintaining test animals on a high-sugar diet during

pregnancy and breast-feeding influences the activity levels of their offspring.

- Beet sugar sensitivity has been reported in medical books. It is not uncommon to have sugar allergies.

- High sugar intake contributes to hypoglycemia and diabetes.

- Consumption of sugars may produce undesirable changes in metabolic risk factors such as blood triglycerides, total cholesterol and uric acid. If consumed with saturated fat, the adverse metabolic effects of the sugars are magnified.

- The factors involved in coronary heart disease are complex, but increased consumption of refined carbohydrate in the form of sugar is a major contributor.

- Richard Wurtman, neurobiologist at MIT, says, "Eating sugar for breakfast could have a particularly dramatic effect on brain composition and behavior."

- At the New York Institute for Child Development, it was shown that a dietary regimen which eliminates sugar has proved to be effective in helping hyperactive children. Improvements are seen in the ability to concentrate, attention spans, irritability, and useless motion.

- Calcium metabolism is linked to sugar metabolism. If you have any problems with insulin—if you are diabetic or hypoglycemic—you will have an exaggerated response of calcium spill when you consume sugar.

- Sugar requires vitamin B6 in order to be metabolized. Vitamin B6 plays a role in magnesium pathways, which in turn affect bone. Furthermore, vitamin B6 helps regulate estrogen levels. So sugar can interfere with bone health plus menstrual and menopausal homeostasis.

- Dr. John Yudkin of England believes that a high sugar intake can be a major contributor to dandruff. Since dandruff is a mild form of seborrheic dermatitis, and B-complex components are an antidote for this condition, the sugar theory makes sense. Sugar requires B vitamins in order to be metabolized. Too much sugar exhausts the B vitamin supply, leaving none to counter the scalp condition.

- Eating sugar with highly refined starches can promote cavities. Jelly or honey on white bread would be an example. The cavity-promoting effect is worse than it would be if eating sugar alone.

Evidence incriminating sugars continues to accumulate. (Knowing some of these facts will be helpful for you as a care-giver, as well as in your own life.)

AFFIRMATIVE ACTION (GENERAL SUGGESTIONS)

Many find that a gradual weaning from sugar is effective.

Don't be fooled by ingredient listings that specify several different kinds of sugar. The manufacturer is allowed to use as many as twelve or more different sweetening agents, and as long as they are not the same, they may be listed separately. This is a ploy to detract from the fact that so much sugar is present in a particular product.

Sugar in cereal is refined sucrose. The sugar in apples is a mixture of fructose, glucose and sucrose, imbedded in a fibrous matrix together with other nutrients designed to accompany the sugars. The insulin and metabolic responses from eating apples and from eating naked sucrose differ greatly.

Sugar has a way of hiding. It is highly absorbent. There is refined sugar in ketchup, some brands of yogurt, juices, instant breakfasts, chewing gum, cough drops, mouthwash, pickles and chewable vitamins.

Don't feel defeated when things get out of control. The cheating incidents will occur with less frequency as the whole family learns a new way of eating. When the body's blood-sugar level drops, the part of the brain that deals with self-control and conscience is altered. That's why so many people say, "Once I eat a piece of fudge, that's it." Biophysical changes can take place which render willpower inoperative.

AFFIRMATIVE ACTION (SPECIFIC SUGGESTIONS)

Use sweet foods to help fill the gap left by the lost love. Try your morning cereal with cinnamon and bananas; sweet potatoes as snacks; pineapple and coconut for dessert; grapes and other fruits in a bowl topped with yogurt and sesame seeds.

Adelle Davis, matriarch of the "New Nutrition" movement, suggests that you advise your children that the family will eat only good food for a week, and that next Saturday you will all indulge in the "other" stuff—all the cola and pie and cakes and candy you can choke down. After a solid week eating only healthful food, most children will get very sick consuming the garbage food. It is too much of a load when they have abstained for a week. Usually they will heave up, get headaches and have royal stomach pains. This is a graphic demonstration of what corrupt food can do. But don't expect this to be a sure-fire solution; sometimes it works and sometimes it doesn't. It is human nature to forget pain and discomfort.

Sugar is a highly refined substance, new to human experience, and totally foreign to the animal kingdom. If sugar were being introduced for sale for the first time, the FDA would probably ban its use because of its correlation with myriad health hazards.

CHANGE #5: HI-Q PROTEIN: QUALITY, NOT QUANTITY

Surely there is a Nobel prize waiting for the researcher who can scientifically demonstrate the exact amount of protein required by human beings. Different theories abound regarding the specifics, but we do know in general that Americans consume too much protein, and that *quality* rather than *quantity* is the critical factor.

As you know, the protein in food is broken down into component parts called amino acids. These individual amino acids are then reassembled in the unique pattern of human protein. You are literally taking something else and converting it into you. Your body doesn't care where the amino acids come from as long as they are present and accounted for in quantities necessary for the restructuring.

A steak may contain protein equal to a quarter of its weight, and an apple may have only a trace of protein. The point is all foods contain some protein, although the amount varies. In addition, the quantities of the individual amino acids differ. When you consume meat, chances are it will give you enough of what you require for the rebuilding. An apple, however, does not supply the necessary quantities of each amino acid. If you need an amino acid missing in your lunch today, but happened to eat a food containing that amino acid yesterday, it's too late. All the amino acids indispensable for creating your new protein must be consumed at the same meal.

More than any other food, with the exception of breast milk, eggs contain amino acids in a pattern closest to that required by humans. There are almost no amino acids left over after the egg's protein is taken apart and rearranged for your use. As for breast milk, it contains only 1 percent protein, but the entire amount is utilized, leaving virtually no amino acids for disposal. A food containing a large percentage of protein does not necessarily yield a large percentage of totally usable amino acids for conversion to human protein.

When you learned that a particular food was a good source of high-quality complete protein, you were taught that this meant that there are enough amino acids for reassembly, with not too many parts left over. But it also indicates that other food values in that food are especially healthful. Fish is such a food. Meat, although a high-protein food, is not in the same category because it is deleterious in other ways. Meat contains high amounts of fat, and it has been shown that Americans who avoid meat have higher bone densities than meat eaters. The more meat included in your diet, the more likely you are to have osteoporosis (porosity of bones) later on; meat eaters lose almost twice as much calcium as their vegetarian friends. The more protein in your diet, the more calcium excreted. Too much protein is not in your best health interest.

Here's the protein content of some foods you may be eating:

1 chicken breast	20.5 grams
2 medium eggs	11.4 grams
6 ounces porterhouse steak	34.3 grams
2 slices bacon	6.4 grams
1 3-ounce can of salmon	23.1 grams
1 tablespoon peanut butter	4.0 grams
1-ounce slice Swiss cheese	8.0 grams

If you are eating bacon and eggs for breakfast, chicken salad for lunch, a peanut butter snack midday, steak for dinner and cheese and crackers while watching TV, you are placing yourself at risk.

We can learn a lot from traditional societies. Other cultures use high-protein foods as embellishments rather than as main ingredients. And there are several techniques that can raise the status of nutrient-dense but protein-poor plant foods so that there will be sufficient quantities of the right amino acids, without burdening the body with too much protein or, as in the case of meat, too much fat. One way is to use legumes—peas, beans or lentils—in which the concentration of protein is high. (Many Asians use this technique by consuming huge quantities of rice.)

You can also combine foods so that the weaknesses of one food are strengthened by the support of another food, a method known as protein complementarity. For example, cereals are poor in the amino acid lysine. But cereals combined with legumes, which contain lysine, provide a mixture of protein that is better than either alone. This health strategy has been known for centuries, despite ignorance of scientific analysis of amino acid profiles. And here is another demonstration of protein complementarity: Many plant foods are weak in methionine. Adding hulled sesame seeds, which have the highest quantity of methionine known, solves the problem.

Few people realize that the high temperatures that go hand in hand with high technology food processing lower amino acid content, thereby reducing the ability to recruit new protein, human style. So once again, primal foods that are minimally processed get the high scores.

PROTEIN COMPLEMENTARITY SUGGESTIONS

Sandwich Spread 4 tablespoons peanut butter; 2 tablespoons sesame butter (tahini); ¼ cup softened butter; 1 tablespoon lemon juice; ½ teaspoon tamari. Blend all ingredients. Makes two or three sandwiches.

Delicious Millet 2 cups water; 1 cup whole millet; dash freshly ground pepper; handful of sunflower seeds; 2 cloves minced garlic. Boil water. Add millet. Lower heat and cook, covered, 15 to 20 minutes or until all water is absorbed. Add pepper, sunflower seeds and garlic. Optional: add raw, diced vegetables. Serves two to four.

Tried-and-True Combos Peanut butter and bread; split pea soup and crackers; rice and beans; tortillas and beans; cereal and sesame seeds; yams and beans.

CHANGE #6: "GETTING FRESH"

Before World War II, commercially prepared foods were produced by the same methods used at home. Today, the foods you buy are the result of very sophisticated technology which could only be duplicated in factories. Products are bleached and blanched, colored and curdled, dampened and dehydrated, emulsified and evaporated, fried, frozen and fabricated, ground and grated, heated and homogenized, mashed, molded, milled and microwaved, pasteurized and pressurized, salted, sweetened and stuffed, or—if we're going from A to Z—in a word, *zapped.*

And guess who pays for all this high tech? Fresh potatoes cost two-thirds less than canned and about 75 percent less than frozen.

But that's not the only cost. Madison Avenue has adeptly implanted a scenario in our minds. Through their skills, we envision beautiful fields of vegetables growing under sunny blue skies. The just-picked products are loaded into bushel baskets at their peak of ripeness, whisked to the nearby plant, and frozen or canned at once. Media hype has us convinced that nutrients have been captured forever in the confines of the packaging, waiting only to be released in your stomach, at your will.

What actually transpires has been expounded by consumer advocates. Destruction of nutrients during heating in canning is dependent on time, temperature and the lability of the nutrient. Over the years, there has been a gradual shift to higher and higher processing temperatures. As an indicator of nutrient losses, note those that occur in the canning of green beans:

Nutrient	Percent of Loss in Canning
Folacin	57.1
Vitamin B6	50.0
Pantothenic acid	60.5
Vitamin A	51.7
Thiamin	62.5
Riboflavin	63.6
Niacin	40.0
Vitamin C	78.9

Additional losses are incurred during storage.

The effects of freeze-preservation on nutrients are also deleterious. Substantial amounts of vitamins and minerals can be lost as a result of many factors, including physical separation (peeling and trimming in preparation for the freezing process), storage (even at correct temperatures), temperature fluctuation and thawing.

In addition to the damage incurred in processing, your body reacts negatively when the form of a food is changed. We have already discussed the effects of eating apples as compared to applesauce and apple juice. This study helps clarify the true meaning of "whole" and "natural." Step #6 on the good health continuum suggests that you discard your can opener, put a lock on your freezer door and consume foods as close to their primal form as possible. In other words, get it fresh, and eat it that way.

At a recent world-wide medical conference, the keynote speaker concluded: "Until our people can enjoy food which is fresh, varied, and unrefined, our health is not likely to improve."

"FRESH" RECIPES

Vegetable Medley. Assorted fresh vegetables; 2 tablespoons vinegar; ½ teaspoon Dijon mustard; freshly ground black pepper. Lightly steam vegetables, placing quicker-cooking vegetables on top of steamer basket—cut in large pieces—(zucchini, broccoli, onions) and slower-cooking vegetables on bottom—cut in smaller pieces—(squash, corn, sweet potatoes). When vegetables reach prime color and are still crisp, remove and cover with mixture of vinegar, mustard and pepper. This rivals any prepared vegetable "convenience" store-bought package. *Nutrition note*: The less steaming, the more nutrient retention.

Carrot, Cabbage and Raisin Salad. 1 cup finely shredded cabbage; 3 cups grated carrots; ½ cup raisins; ½ cup sunflower/yogurt dressing (see below); 2 teaspoons lemon juice. Mix vegetables and raisins. Add mayonnaise and lemon juice. Stir well. *Nutrition note*: Soak raisins for two hours to rehydrate before adding to salad.

Sunflower/Yogurt Dressing. 1 cup sunflower seeds; 1 cup plain yogurt; 2 tablespoons chopped onions; 2 tablespoons chopped celery; 1 tablespoon dill. Blend all ingredients. *Nutrition note*: Sprout sunflower seeds for one day before use.

CHANGE #7: HOW TO SHOP FOR YOUR FAT

There are no ingredient listings on chocolate-dipped strawberries, or slices of apple pie purchased in the bake shop, or on the bag of take-out french fries. There should be ingredient listings, and they should read: *Contains free radicals. The Surgeon General says this may be dangerous to your health.*

FAT FACTS

Fat has received bad press, but you know that we cannot survive without fatty acids. The body requires fatty acids in its daily biochemical activity, but it is unable to make them by its own chemical processes. You may recall learning that your body can make all the parts of the fat molecules except for polyunsaturated fatty acids, called PUFAs.

PUFAs are found in naturally occurring vegetable and fish oils, and in human milk. All you require is about a teaspoonful a day, but believe it or not, it is hard to find good, unprocessed oil.

PUFAs are very chemically reactive. Because they are so reactive, they are affected by improper storage, and become rancid very easily. Early rancidity of fat is not detectable by smell or taste. When you eat foods that have gone rancid, they interfere with the usefulness of PUFAs in your body.

Fat molecules are large and complex, and they have a specific configuration in space—a physical form. When we look at a glove, we recognize that it was designed to fit a hand, but we also know that there are right-hand and left-hand gloves, and that one doesn't fit the other. They are mirror images, alike but not identical because they are reversed. Chemical molecular structures are also capable of having mirror-image forms. Your body can use only the so-called cis form of fatty acids. That's the one that fits into your body machinery; in fact, it fits like a glove! But here's the rub: when fats are commercially processed, we convert some of the cis fatty acids into trans configurations. And these trans fatty acids do not fit into the body machinery. Now you're trying to put the right-hand glove on the left hand, and this gums up the works.

All processed fats have this unhealthful form of fatty acid. For example, there is probably no healthful margarine available in the United States. Most, if not all, cooking oils and fats contain excessive quantities of trans fatty acids.

One of the most important factors triggering rancidity in fat is exposure to excessive heat. PUFA-rich oils may be used for cooking, but only at low heat and for short cooking times. These oils, once opened, should be kept refrigerated, and used promptly. If not used in four months, they should be discarded and replaced. Typical oils high in PUFAs include safflower, sunflower and sesame.

Let us assume you've abided by *change #7,* and you have taken your PUFAs from healthful food sources rather than overprocessed, damaged foodstuffs. Now your body has to convert the oil into a usable form. If you don't have enough vitamin C, or you are deficient in vitamin B6, or if you are overweight, have diabetes or you are a senior citizen, or you have too many trans fatty acids in your diet, chances are you will have difficulty converting vegetable oils for body use. Because of the extreme importance of the need for PUFAs, supplementation with already-converted oils is recommended.

Gamma-linolenic acid (GLA) is the converted form of fatty acids. GLA is not found in too many foods. Fortunately, one or two plant foods in which it does occur have been used to produce excellent supplements. Among them is the black currant seed. Besides GLA, black currant seeds contain other oils that provide a balanced blend that enable you to meet all requirements of these nutrients, essential for your body's normal physiological needs.

So suggestion #7 is to beware of processed oils and specialty gourmet foods made with them, and to try to get the fat components of your diet from the primal food source itself, with some supplementation to help things along.

OIL-FREE SALAD DRESSINGS

Tofu/Sesame Dressing. 1 cup tofu; 1 cup water; 2 tablespoons tamari; ¼ cup sesame butter (ground sesame seeds); 1 tablespoon chopped parsley; 2 to 3 cloves garlic; ½ cup lemon juice; 1 teaspoon kelp. Blend all ingredients.

Caraway Dressing. 1 avocado; 1 tomato; juice of 1 lemon; 1 tablespoon caraway seeds; 2 cloves garlic; 1 tablespoon kelp. Blend all ingredients.

Avocado Special. 1 avocado; ¼ cup fresh chopped comfrey; 2 cloves garlic; small amount of carrot or beet juice. Blend all ingredients.

Fruit/Nut Dressing. 2 cups apple juice; ½ cup almonds; 1 cup fresh pitted cherries. Blend all ingredients.

Herb Dressing. ¼ cup chopped celery; ½ cup green pepper; 2 cloves garlic; 1½ cup chopped onion; 2 cups tomatoes; ½ teaspoon basil; ½ teaspoon oregano; pinch of thyme; water to blend. Blend all ingredients. Allow mixture to sit for 8 hours. Add chunks of any fresh vegetables if desired.

CHANGE #8: CULTURE—OUTSIDE IN: GOOD-GUY BACTERIA

A study of the history of medicine reveals that it takes about 80 years for a discovery to be accepted and put into everyday practice. This has been true of almost all great medical disclosures.

Lactobacillic-fermented foods have been used for ages, but the pioneering work that established the reasons for their benefits dates back only to 1908. It is no surprise, then, that the popularity of acidophilus has only recently come to the fore. Physicians are now prescribing it for many patients and for many reasons.

THE "CULTURAL" ADVANTAGES

The researcher who first identified the advantageous bacteria noted that Bulgarians who ate yogurt were living long lives. Several new studies have confirmed that lactobacilli used in the fermentation process may improve the nutritional quality as well as the nutritional quantity of cultured products by increasing the B-vitamin and enzyme contents. It also improves both the biological value and the availability of essential amino acids, the building blocks of protein. In addition, during fermentation the lactobacilli can produce natural antibiotics, natural anticarcinogenic compounds, natural anticholesteremic compounds, and even compounds which retard or inactivate toxins and poisons. This information was revealed at a worldwide symposium of the Swedish Nutrition Foundation.

The anticholesteremic effects were discovered in 1979. Supplementation of the diet with acidophilus resulted in decreased cholesterol levels. In 1978 the Russians reported the favorable use of kumiss (a fermented milk drink made from mare's milk) in the treatment of a number of diseases including chronic lung disease, digestive tract disease and myocardial infarction. Yet another study demonstrated antitumor activity. (Feeding patients milk, lactose, lactic acid or cells killed by heat did not show any inhibitory effect.) Certain strains of lactobacilli have been shown to degrade nitrosamines, the converted and carcinogenic form of nitrates and nitrites.

A healthy intestinal gut is populated with an assemblage of good-guy bacteria, which crowds out bacteria of disreputable lineage. You can resist enemy invasion by entrenching your normal flora with good-guy sentries.

FERMENTED FOODS

Nearly every civilization has consumed cultured milk of one type or another. Fermentation with lactic acid bacteria is one of humankind's oldest methods of food processing and food preservation. Long ago the process was initiated by organisms present in the raw foods, in the air or on utensils. Obviously this made the production slow and very unpredictable. High technology has promoted the use of specific starter cultures and very precise conditions of time, temperature and so on. This results in not only a superior product, but one which insures microbial safety.

The experts are no longer saying, *You are what you eat.* They are now saying, *You are what you assimilate.* The best food in the world is of no value if its nutrients are not digested and assimilated. A cultured product has the same caloric value as the food from which it has been made, but it is more nutritious because the major food constituents (proteins, fats and carbohydrates) may be predigested. It has been demonstrated, for example, that yogurt has a higher digestibility and higher biological value than the milk from which it has been prepared. An Indian fermented cereal known as Idli has a 33 percent increased protein efficiency rate compared to the unfermented product.

Another study shows that the higher nutritional values of cultured products translate into improved physical performance when these foods are ingested.

What kind of fermented foods are eaten today? Fermented sausages made from the meat of a variety of animals and fish are consumed worldwide. Fermented vegetables (which were originated by the Chinese as a preservation method) are now an important part of the diet of Far Eastern peoples, Europeans and even Americans. Yogurt, cheese, kefir, kumiss, pickles, sauerkraut, yeast bread and tempeh are examples of fermented foods. Cultured products have been, and still are, of extreme importance in the nutrition of people throughout the world. The nutritional advantages of cultured vegetable and dairy products, however, exceed by far those of cultured meat products.

An antinutritional factor in soybeans is totally eliminated when they are fermented. The same is true of the undesirable phytates found in the outer husk of grains (such as wheat bran). An added advantage is that the flatulent effect of beans is destroyed if they are fermented. Good news for the allergic and migraine-headache sufferers: the use of lactic starter cultures prevents the production of histamine and tyramine in several food products. Chances are you will be hearing more about this in the near future.

So suggestion #8 is to allow viable acidophilus bacteria to set up housekeeping in your intestine, creating an ecological system that will help you absorb nutrients and create new ones, and, in general, serve to increase your wellbeing. (See specific suggestions for supplementing with acidophilus cultures in Chapter 5.)

CHANGE #9: FROM SEED TO SALAD—HOW TO SPROUT

Sprouting may have the reputation of being esoteric, "way out." If you eat sprouts, you run the risk of being labeled a health nut. But there is no better way to beat the establishment while procuring more healthful foods.

If you combined half a dozen sprouts (alfalfa, mung, radish, azuki, sunflower and lentils are possibilities), added herb seasonings, a dash of apple cider vinegar (remember how good this is for your bones), a few slices of avocado, and enjoyed the medley for lunch with a chunk of sprouted grain bread, the cost of the sprout salad potpourri would be less than fifty cents.

SPROUTING EQUIPMENT

The best equipment for sprouting is the one-quart canning jar. These jars are widemouthed, withstand boiling water for thorough cleansing, and are quite durable. They range in cost from one to three dollars each, depending on whether you are shopping in a bargain basement or a major department store. Discard the glass tops, rubber rings and metal wires. All you need is the jar.

Buy nylon mosquito netting at a hardware store, and dig out some short, thick rubberbands. (You must have some in that "catchall" drawer in the kitchen.) Cut the netting into squares large enough to cover the tops of the jars, with enough of a flap to secure with the rubberbands. This is the best and cheapest sprouting equipment available.

SPROUTING INSTRUCTIONS

Soak each variety of seeds or beans in one cup of water in a jar overnight. It is preferable to use pure spring water for the soaking procedure. Recommended quantities:

alfalfa	one tablespoon
mung	two tablespoons
radish	one-half tablespoon
azuki	two tablespoons
chick peas	three tablespoons
lentils	two tablespoons
sunflower seeds	two tablespoons
soybeans	one tablespoon
wheatberries	two tablespoons
buckwheat	two tablespoons
clover	one tablespoon
rye	one tablespoon
sesame	one tablespoon

In the morning, pour the water off. (Use this water for your plants—they'll love it! Or save the water to use as stock.) Dumping the seeds into a strainer facilitates the washing process. Rinse thoroughly under the faucet. Return seeds to jar after shaking strainer by tapping against side of sink. Cover jar with mesh netting and tight rubberband.

Place jar upside down at a slight angle in a dish rack, so that the remaining water can run off. Sprouts appreciate moisture, but not puddles. Rinse seeds again in the evening. If you can rinse them again in the middle of the day, that's an advantage. Now that the seeds are no longer soaking in water, they can be rinsed directly under the faucet in the jars. The mesh netting, held in place with the rubberband, prevents the seeds from escaping when the water is poured off. (Be sure the rubberband is tight enough.)

Many people start the procedure in the dark because this expedites growth. You may find, however, that when you hide the jars in a closet, you forget about them. When you unveil them a week or so later, you will find something not unlike Pandora's box. Another possibility is to place the jar in a paper bag and leave it on the kitchen counter as a reminder. We skip this procedure because sprouts which germinate in daylight develop with more nutrients.

Seeds may be consumed at any stage of sprouting, but harvesting at their peak offers the most nutritional value. Vitamin C is synthesized during germination, and the concentrations of some of the B vitamins is also increased, along with other nutrients. The peak germination times for the most popular seeds are: alfalfa, 4 days; mung, 3 days; radish, 4 days; azuki, 2 days; chick-peas, 1 day; lentils, 2 days; sunflower seeds, 1 day; soybeans, 1 or 2 days; wheatberries, 2 or 3 days; buckwheat, 3 or 4 days; clover, 4 days; rye, 2 days; sesame, 1 or 2 days.

Since seeds and environments vary, it is advisable to experiment, using a good sprouting book as a guide. Alfalfa, mung and garbanzo beans are excellent sprouts for beginners. Before consuming, leave sprouts in indirect sunlight. This will "green" the leaves, adding chlorophyll.

Refrigerated sprouts last up to a week. But since they are growing in your kitchen, the "farm" couldn't be any closer. It is best to "harvest" as needed to optimize nutrient value. Sprouts are so inexpensive that we discard rather than save any surplus. (For the novice, "harvesting" sprouts simply means taking them from the jar.)

You may want to introduce the technique of sprouting to patients who are going to be hospitalized for a long time, and have little energy. (That's all it takes to get involved in this kind of project.) The patient's involvement throughout any healing process makes care activities more successful. (Can you envision sprouting jars lining hospital window sills?)

SPROUT RECIPES

Tossed Green Salad with Sprouts. Romaine lettuce; sprigs of watercress; 1 onion, sliced thin; 1 cup alfalfa sprouts; 1 shredded carrot; ¼ cup chopped parsley; ⅛ cup sprouted sunflower seeds. *Nutrition tip*: Watercress is so named because it grows in water and contains minerals found in marine vegetables. Serves two as main course, four if side dish.

Wheatberry Balls. ½ cup cream cheese; 1 cup sprouted wheatberries; 1 cup chopped nuts; 1 cup raisins; toasted sesame seeds. Mix all ingredients except sesame seeds until blended. Shape into small balls; roll in toasted sesame seeds. (Makes about 24 balls.) *Nutrition tip*: Cream cheese has the best calcium/phosphorus ratio of all the popular cheeses. Makes about twenty-four balls.

Mung Bean Salad. 1 cup mung bean sprouts; 1 cup finely chopped celery; 1 cup grated carrots; ½ cup chopped pine nuts; 1 tablespoon sesame seeds; leafy green lettuce. Combine sprouts, celery, grated carrots, nuts and sesame seeds. Serve on lettuce with sesame dressing. *Nutrition tips*: Grated carrots are excellent for constipation. Serves four.

Sesame Dressing. ¼ cup ground sesame seeds; ½ cup water; 2 tablespoons lemon juice; ½ clove garlic, crushed. Blend all until smooth. *Nutrition tip*: Purchase mechanically hulled sesame seeds. Unhulled seeds are too high in oxalic acid (which binds calcium) and chemically hulled seeds have chemical residues.

Sauteed Sprouts. 2 tablespoons sesame oil; 1 large onion, sliced thin; 4 cups mung bean sprouts; 1 tablespoon tamari. Heat skillet over medium heat. Add oil and onion; sauté 5 minutes. Add mung bean sprouts; sauté until heated through. Season with tamari. *Nutrition tips*: Sesame oil is a very stable oil because it has a built-in antioxidant. Serves four.

You can also make sprout omelets, add the sprouts to sandwich fillings, use them as snacks, simmer them with fish and drop them into soups.

The process of germination induces an increase in nutrient content. Anything that can grow into a plant or an animal must obviously have a select store of power. Sprouting leads to the manufacture of new protein, sugars and fats within the growing seed. Using a variety of sprouts can supply *complete* protein, to say nothing of the vitamin and mineral values. We sincerely hope you will take the time to learn to sprout. Once you know what you're doing, you need spend no more than ten minutes in the morning and ten minutes at night. Not enough to be a burden; just enough to give you pleasure and very special immune-building nutrients. Again—what a wonderful healing tool for patients!

Summing up

Most people are amazed at how quickly they reach a new level of wellness when they begin to modify their diets, even if they were not "sick" initially. Feeling better or being less sick acts as its own reward and encourages continued shifting.

In conclusion, you should remember that the secret of good health is so simple, it's right under your nose: it's your mouth.

EPILOGUE

A Swedish physician pointed out that the word for food in Swedish is *livsmedel*, which, when translated directly, means life or life remedy. He went on to say that many products are called *food* when in fact they should actually be called *death*, because they promote sickness and hasten death.

If good food is medicine, as Hippocrates maintained, we have a medicine that is completely nontoxic and without side effects when given in optimal doses. All types of diseases can develop from lack of common foods: lack of protein, lack of water, lack of salt and so on. The other side of the coin is that all types of diseases can develop from an overdose of the same substances: too much protein, too much salt and even too much water.

Summary specifics for optimal health and healing

Based on clinical experience at The Stress Center in Huntington, Long Island, New York, we discovered that "optimal diet" could alleviate varied and sundry symptoms, mild or intense. Those who followed its tenets not only began to be free of symptoms, but looked incredibly younger.

"My internist told me that my multiple sclerosis was something I had to live with. He says it's pure coincidence that I look and feel so much better. I cannot convince him that it's the diet change."

"You mean it was that simple? I've been taking stool softeners for twenty years, since age thirteen, and in three weeks my problem has disappeared."

"For the first time in my life I have color in my face."

"For the first time in years I don't need an antacid after every meal."

These are just a few of several hundred comments typical of those heard by nutritionists day after day. As for the tempo at which a person makes the changes, there are surprises. Some people don't want to get well—ever. Others with serious degenerative disease can only alter things slowly, even when more rapid modifications might mean quicker recovery. Those who give you the impression that you are wasting both your time and theirs during an initial counseling session, may report that they have, after all, made changes. Personality and nutrition awareness, rather than degree of illness, dictate how receptive people are to turning things around.

Optimal diet appears stringent at first glance. But volumes have been filled with endless varieties of recipes based on the accepted foods. Optimal diet follows.

You should *not* eat or drink Milk (whole), milk (skim or low fat), half-and-half, tea, coffee, decaf, tap water, cheese and other milk products, fruit juice, head or iceberg lettuce, salt butter, margarine, dried fruit, citrus fruit, ice cream, pretzels, canned soup, potato chips, wheat products, wheat germ, bran, white bread, white rice, supermarket whole wheat bread, bottled oils, nuts purchased without shells (unless sprouted), cola, diet soda, cake, cookies, crackers, canned or frozen anything, sugar, salt, honey, processed flour.

What's left?

You *can* eat Eggs (fertile only; poached, boiled, or sunny-side-up are best); sweet butter (in very small amounts); these whole grains: millet, brown rice, buckwheat (without milk; use yogurt or cinnamon); Essene bread (made from sprouted grains); small amount of viable yogurt or acidophilus with each meal; cold-water fish (eat the skin too).

You *must* eat Vegetables, every day, a lot. Raw. Lightly steamed. As much as the appetite and digestion tolerate. You cannot overdose on vegetables. Leafy greens: parsley, watercress, Bibb or romaine lettuce, etc.

You can also eat Fruit in moderation (fruit formula: 1 fruit to 3 portions of vegetables); condiments (all unprocessed kinds—onions and garlic especially).

You should eat foods to reduce toxic levels 1 cup peas or beans daily, 1 cup alfalfa sprouts daily, lots of raw vegetables.

Beverages If herb teas are unpalatable, add unprocessed apple juice until taste buds are reeducated. Diminish juice until it is no longer needed. Add cinnamon or cinnamon stick to herb tea. Drink lots of water (pure, of course).

Some people respond to the diet changes immediately. Others require several months before feeling better. There are those who even feel worse before improving. But there is a pot of gold at the end of this rainbow.

Nutrition education

PERIODICALS RECOMMENDED BY E. LYNN FRALEY, R.N., DR. P.H.
New England Journal of Medicine
American Journal of Clinical Nutrition
Lancet
Nutrition Reviews
American Journal of Nursing
Nursing Research
Western Journal of Nursing Research

BOOKS

Independent Nursing Intervention, Mariah Snyder. New York: John Wiley & Sons, 1985.

The Physicians' Drug Manual: Prescription and Nonprescription Drugs, Rubin Bressler et al. Garden City, New York: Doubleday & Co., 1981.

Self-Care Nursing: Theory and Practice, Nancy J. Steiger and Juliene G. Lipsom. Bowie, Maryland: Brady Communications Co., 1985.

FILM STRIPS

From Encore Visual Education, Inc.
1235 South Victory Blvd.
Burbank, CA 91502
Telephone: 213-843-6515
  Filmstrips available:

Beans, Beans, Beans
Fruitful Menu
Grain Cookery
Vegetarianism
Food: The Choice is Yours
The Tofu Experience
Kitchen With a Mission: Nutrition
The Seed Sprout Secret
The Peanut Butter

From Bergwall Productions
839 Steward Ave.
P.O. Box 238
Garden City, NY 11520
Telephone: 800-645-3565
   Filmstrips available:
   Exploding Nutrition Myths, Part I
      The Food-Group Foolers
      The Protein Picture
      The Milky Way
      Give Produce Priority
      Striking Oil
      The Grain Robbery
   Exploding Nutrition Myths, Part II
      Dietary Goals
      The Sad State of Overweight
      Complex Carbohydrates Simplified
      Sugar: Not Such Sweet Talk
      Cut the Fat
      The Salt Shake-Up
      Beyond the New Health Horizon

INDEX

Absorption, of nutrients, 71–72, 78, 136
Acetylcholine, stress and need for, 142
Acidophilus
 carrot-grown, 100
 and colon cancer, 110
 "good" bacteria, 196
 health advantages, 195
 and infection, 115
 and nutrient absorption, 73
ACTH. *See* Adrenocorticotrophic hormone
Additives. *See* Food additives
Adrenalin, in stress reaction, 131, 135
Adrenocorticotrophic hormone (ACTH), 145
Aging
 and GLA, 99
 and stress, 137
Alcoholism, 124
 and GLA, 99
Alfalfa, 113
Algae, 100
Aloe vera, as anesthetic, 103
Allergens, common food, 126–127
Allergy, 126–127
 and arthritis, 109
Amino acids
 and cholesterol, 113

deficiencies, 107
digestion of, 135
and protein, 186–187, 188
Aminosalicylic acid, and timing of meals, 85
Analgesics, and vitamin C, 83
Anemia
 and dilantin, 78
 and phenytoin, 78
Antacids, and water-soluble vitamins, 83
Antibiotics
 and B vitamins, 70
 and fat-soluble vitamins, 82
 and soda, 86
Anticoagulants
 and vitamin E, 83
 and vitamin K, 87
Anticonvulsants, and vitamin D, 83
Antidepressants
 and vitamin B6, 84
 and vitamin C, 83
Antigens
 and acidophilus, 73
 food as, 72
Antigout medication, and vitamin B12, 84
Antihistamines, and soda, 86
Antihypertensives, and vitamin B6, 84

Antimicrobials
  and folic acid, 85
  and steatorrhea, 85
  and vitamin B12, 85
Antinutrients, 92
Antioxidants
  benefits of, 95–96
  and toxins, 112
  vitamin E as, 102
Apple, ingestion of various forms, 61–62
Apresoline, 79
  and vitamin B6, 84
Arginine, 113
Arsenic, 43–44
Arthritis. See Rheumatoid arthritis
Ascorbic acid. See also Vitamin C
  and glucocorticoids, 84
  stress and need for, 142–143
  and sulfa drugs, 83–84
  in wound healing, 102
Aspirin, and vitamin C, 79, 81, 108
Assimilation, importance, 72, 196–197
Atherosclerosis, and alfalfa, 113
Azulfidine, 80

Baking soda, and thiamin, 70
Belladonna, and gastric acid, 85
Beta-carotene, and cancer, 110
Bioflavonoids, 14–15
Biotin, 23
Birth control pills, nutritional regimen for users, 103
Blood pressure
  and calcium, 113
  and GLA, 99
  and sugar, 182
Bran, and manganese, 70
Breathing exercises, prior to surgery, 102
Buckwheat, 177–178, 179
Burn-out syndrome, 133
Burns
  calorie intake, 121
  fluid intake, 122, 123
  high-protein diet for, 122, 123
  and vitamin C, 121–122, 123
  vitamin supplementation, 122
  and zinc, 123–124

Cadmium
  and high blood pressure, 112
  and zinc, 112
Caffeine
  and aspirin, 86
  and fatigue, 86
  and heart disease, 86
  and iron absorption, 69
  and nicotine, 86
Calcium, 26–27
  and blood pressure, 113
  deficiency, 107
  and high-fat diet, 69
  and magnesium, 88
  and osteoporosis, 118, 119–120
  and sugar, 183
  and vitamin D, 88
Calories, 62–63
Cancer
  and acidophilus, 110
  and fat in diet, 109–110
  and manganese, 110
  and selenium, 110
  stress as factor in, 139
  and vitamins C and E, 110
  and weight loss, 111
  and zinc, 110
Canning, loss of nutrients in, 190
Carbohydrates, refined, 62
Carcinogens
  and antioxidants, 95–96
  and well-balanced diet, 89
Carodophilus, 100
Carnitine, and blood triglycerides, 114
Cells
  nutrition for, 107–108
  oxidation process, 4
  T. See T-cells

Chemotherapy
  nausea and vomiting, 111
  vitamin-drug balance, 84
  vitamins C and E, 110
Chlorella, 100
Cholesterol
  and alfalfa, 113
  and GLA, 99
  lowering, 112–114
  and soybean-rich diet, 113
  and surfactants, 82
Cholestyramine, and nutrient absorption, 79, 82
Choline, 25–26
  and methionine, 1
Chromium, 36
  and American diet, 70
  and diabetes, 116
  and HDL, 114
  stress, effects on, 144
Clofibrate, and nutrient absorption, 82
Cobalamin, 20–21, 84
Codeine, and soda, 86
Coffee, 86
  and heart disease, 114
  prior to surgery, 101
Colbenemid, and vitamin B12, 84
Colchicine, 79, 84
Collagen, production and stress, 138
Constipation
  contributory factors, 125
  foods to eradicate, 125–126
Copper, 34–35
Cortisone, and vitamin C, 83
Coumadin
  and vitamin B12, 84
  and vitamin C, 83
  and vitamin E, 83
Crohn's disease, 118
Cultured food, 196–197
Cuprimine, 79
Cystine, and methionine, 1

Dandruff, and sugar, 184

Depression, serotonin levels in, 143
Diabetes
  and alcohol, 116–117
  and chromium, 116
  and diet, 115, 116, 117
  and exercise, 117
  and inositol, 116
  and vitamin A, 82
Diagnosis, medical field emphasis on, 106–107
Diet, 64
  and heart disease, 112–114
  four-food-group, 66–67
  high-fat, 69
  high-fiber, 88
  high-protein, 69
  low-fat, 112, 114
  meat-free, 112
  optimal, 73, 203–204
  postoperative, 101
  pre-operative, 101–102
  soybean-rich, 113
Digestion, 71
  process, 135–136
  stress, effect on, 130–131, 134–135, 136, 138
Dilantin
  and folate levels, 78
  and vitamin D, 83
Dioctyl sodium sulfosuccinate
  and cholesterol, 82
  and vitamin A, 82
Disease, resistance to, 137
Diuretics
  and potassium, 113
  and water-soluble vitamins, 83
Doriden, and vitamin D, 79, 83
Drug abuse, 124
Drugs. See also individual drugs
  body's reaction to, 81
  and increased nutrient needs, 81
  individual reactions to, 86
  multiple actions of, 80
  and nutrient interactions, 78–87

Drugs *(continued)*
  and side effects, 80–81

Eggs, and cholesterol, 112
Elavil, and vitamin B6 (pyridoxine), 84
Endorphins, 137–138
Energy, 2
Enzymes
  and nutrients, 3–4
  and vitamins, 3–4
Erythromycin, and gastric acid, 85
Essential fatty acids (EFA), 96–97
Estrogens
  and folic acid absorption, 84–85
  and vitamin B6 (pyridoxine), 84
Exercise
  in diabetes, 117
  as stress reducer, 146–147

Fat
  in American diet, 109
  and cancer, 109–110
  processed, 109–110, 112
  saturated, 65, 99
  unsaturated, 65, 69, 99
Fatty acids
  as energy, 136
  essential (EFAs), 96–97
  Omega-3. *See* Omega-3 fatty acids
  Omega-6, 98–99
  polyunsaturated. *See* Polyunsaturated fatty acids
  and stress, 138–139
Fermented foods, 197
Fiber, and satiety, 62
Fibrocystic disease, and GLA, 99
Fluorine, 39
Folic acid, 22
  and antimicrobials, 85
  and chemotherapy, 84
  and food storage, 70
  and seizures, 78–79
Food
  antigen-antibody reactions to, 72
  contaminated, 52–53
  hospital. *See* Hospital food
  nutrient value, 69–70
Food additives, 65, 66, 67
Food processing
  nutrient losses and, 53
  potassium-to-sodium ratio in, 145
Four-food-group diet, 66–67
Free radical pathology, 95
Frozen foods, 67–68, 70, 190

Gamma-linolenic acid (GLA)
  to meet body's fatty acid needs, 193–194
  role of, 98–99
Gantrisin, and ascorbic acid, 83–84
Ginseng, 120
GLA. *See* Gamma-linolenic acid
Glucocorticoids
  and calcium absorption, 84
  and phosphorus absorption, 81
  and vitamin D, 84
Glucose, 4
  level of, and nutrition, 115–117
  source of energy, 136
Glutethimide, and vitamin D, 79, 83
Grains, adding to diet, 176–181
Griseofulvin, and high-fat meals, 85

Heart disease
  and diet, 112–114
  and stress, 138
Hegsted, Mark, 73
Hexachlorophene, 78
Hospital food. *See also* Institutional cooking
  liabilities of, 46–49, 63, 121

Hydralazine, 79
Hydration, prior to surgery, 102
Hyperlipidemia, 117
Hyperthyroid metabolism, and vitamin A, 82
Hypoglycemia, 115, 117
Hypothalamus, and stress effect, 131–132, 134

Imagery, as relaxation technique, 56
Immune system, and digestion/assimilation, 72–73
Immunocompetence, and nutritional deficiency, 63
Indocin, and vitamin C, 83
Infection, and nutrition, 114–115
Ingestion, 70–71
Inositol, 24
 and diabetes, 116
 tranquilizing effect of, 146
Insomnia, relaxation technique for, 59
Institutional cooking
 family take-ins as alternative, 156–158
 nurse's influence on, 152–155, 158–163
 and nutrition, 149–152
Iodine, 39–40
Iron, 32
 absorption, 69
 and cholesterol-lowering drugs, 82
 and stress, 144
 and vitamin C, 88, 123
 and vitamin E, 83
Isoniazid, and vitamin B6 (pyridoxine), 84

Kaochlor, and vitamin B12, 84
Kaufman, William, 109
Kayciel, 80
Kryptopyrrole, 143

Lactobacillus bulgaricus, 101

Laxatives
 effects of regular use, 82
 and vitamin D, 83
Lecithin, and cholesterol, 112
Loneliness, 139
Lysine, 113

Magnesium, 28
 and calcium, 88
 stress and reduction of, 144
Malnutrition
 and American diet, 69
 causes of, 52–54
 drug-induced, 77
 and hospitalization, 47–48, 49, 53–54
 symptoms, 49–52
Manganese, 35–36
 and bran, 70
 and cancer, 110
Meat, as source of nutrition, 187
Medication. *See* Drugs
Methionine
 and choline, 1
 and cystine, 1
Methotrexate, detoxification with vitamins, 84
Milk, 121
 nutritional problems, 121
 sour, benefits of, 101
Millet, 178, 179
Mineral oil, 79
 effects of regular use, 82
Minerals, 6–7
 arsenic, 43–44
 calcium, 26–27
 chelated, 96
 chromium, 36
 competition between, 70
 copper, 34–35
 deficiencies, 50–51
 fluorine, 39
 and high-fiber diets, 88
 iodine, 39–40
 iron, 32
 magnesium, 28

Minerals *(continued)*
  manganese, 35–36
  molybdenum, 40–41
  nickel, 42–43
  phosphorus, 29
  potassium, 30
  selenium, 37
  silicon, 38
  sodium, 31
  trace elements, 96
  vanadium, 41–42
  zinc, 33–34
Molybdenum, 40–41
Monoamine oxidase inhibitors, and tyramine-containing foods, 87
Mononucleosis, 139
Mycifradin, 79

Neomycin, 79
  and fat-soluble vitamins, 85
  and folic acid, 85
  and steatorrhea, 85
  and vitamin B12, 79, 85
Niacin, 17–18
  and cholesterol, 111
  and stress, 146
Niacinamide, quieting effect, 146
Nickel, 42–43
Nicotine
  and caffeine, 86
  and drug interactions, 86
Nitrates, and vitamin C, 96
Nitrofurantoin, and timing of meals, 85
Nitrosamines, 96
Noise, and hospital patients, 58–59
Nourishment, 64
Nurses
  job-related risks, 166–167
  personal nutrition, 167–168
Nutrient-dense foods, 69–70
Nutrients
  absorption of, 136
  with calming effects, 146
  chart, 9–44
  and drug interactions, 78–87
  and enzymes, 3–4
  interdependence of, 4, 6–7
  loss of in food processing, 53
  patient needs, 48–49, 61
  and processed foods, 64–69
  utilization, 7–8, 71
  in wound healing, 102
Nutrition, 64
  "balanced," 64–69
  hospital, nurse's influence on, 74–75, 152–155, 158–163
  and immune function, 102, 105
  and institutional cooking, 149–152
  optimal, 92, 93
  personal, steps for changing, 169–202
Nutritional deficiency, 63

Oats, 177, 180
Omega-3 fatty acids, 97–98
  and cholesterol levels, 112–113
Omega-6 fatty acids, 98–99
Opiates, and stress, 138
Optimal diet, 73, 203–204
Oral contraceptives, and nutrient absorption, 84–85
Osteoporosis, 117–118
  and antioxidants, 119
  and calcium, 118, 119–120
  and chlorella, 120
  and exercise, 120
  and ginseng, 120
  and glucocorticoids, 84, 118
  and organ meats, 119
  and processed foods, 120
  and refined sugar, 120
  and sunbaths, 118
  and vitamin D, 118–119

PABA, 25
Pantothenic acid, 18–19
  and stress, 144, 146

Para-aminobenzoic acid. *See* PABA
Parasympathetic nervous system, 132–133, 135
Pectin, and blood sugar, 115
Penicillamine, 79
  and vitamin B6 (pyridoxine), 84
Penicillin, and fat-soluble vitamins, 82
Penicillin G, and gastric acid, 85
Phenobarbital, and vitamin D, 83
Phenylalanine, and tyrosine, 1
Phenylbutazone, and timing of meals, 85
Phenytoin, and folate levels, 78
Phosphorus, 29
  and high-fat diet, 69
Pill. *See* Birth control pills
Platelet aggregation, reduction of, 113
Polyunsaturated fatty acids (PUFAs)
  cis/trans configurations, 192–193
  difficulty getting, 192–193
  GLA, supplementation with, 193
  and prostaglandin production, 98–99
Potassium, 30
  and diuretics, 113
Potassium chloride, 80
Potassium supplements, and vitamin B12, 84
Premarin, and vitamin B6, 84
Propantheline, and gastric acid, 85
Prostaglandins, 98
Protein, 186–189
Pyridoxine, 19–20, 84

Questran, and nutrient absorption, 79, 82

Radiation therapy, effects of, 110–111

Recipes
  grains/breads/cereals, 179–181
  high-protein, 188–189
  salad dressing/sauce, 176, 194
  salt substitutes, 175
  snacks, 171–172
  sprouts, 201–202
  vegetables, 191
Recommended Daily Allowances (RDAs), 8, 69, 92–93
Refined carbohydrates, digestion of, 62
Relaxation, techniques for, 56–59
Rheumatoid arthritis
  and exercise, 109
  and food allergy, 109
  and niacin, 109
  and pantothenic acid, 109
  and vitamin B6, 108
  and vitamin D, 108
  zinc and copper balance, 109
Riboflavin, 16–17
  and chemotherapy, 84
Rice, 178, 179
Rifamate, and vitamin B6 (pyridoxine), 84

Salicylates, 80
  and folate, 79
  and vitamin C, 79
Salt
  alternatives to, 172–176
  and heart disease, 113
Sauna, as therapy, 102
Scarring, and vitamin E, 102–103
Scleroderma, and GLA, 99
Seizures, and folic acid, 78–79
Selenium, 37
  and cancer, 110
  deficiency, 70
Selye, Hans, 137
Senior citizen(s), and nutrient-drug interactions, 87–88
Serotonin, and depression, 143
Sesame seeds, 123

Index

Silicon, 38
Smoking, prior to surgery, 101
Snacks, changing to healthful, 169–172
Soda
  and antibiotics, 86
  and antihistamines, 86
  and codeine, 86
Sodium, 31
  and drinking water, 87
Soft drinks. *See* Soda
Sprouts
  how to grow, 198–200
  nutritional value, 202
  recipes, 201–202
Steroids, and vitamin C, 83
Stress
  acetylcholine, need for, 142
  ACTH, role of, 145
  allergic responses, 139
  ascorbic acid, need for, 142–143
  and cancer, 139
  chromium deficiency, 144
  and collagen production, 138
  and dental caries, 139
  effect on digestion, 130–131, 134–135
  and endorphins, 137–138
  exercise, importance of, 146–147
  and fatty acid levels, 138–139
  and heart disease, 138
  of hospital environment, 133
  hypothalamus, role of, 131–132, 134, 141
  imagery technique for, 56–57
  and immunoglobin secretion rate, 139
  and iron, 144
  and isolation, 139
  magnesium, effect of, 144
  and malnourishment, 145
  and mononucleosis, 139
  pantothenic acid, role of, 144, 146
  patient, signs of, 54–55
  physiology of, 131–135
  potassium-to-sodium ratio under, 145
  relaxation techniques, 57–58
  serotonin precursors and depression, 143
  sympathetic nervous system and, 132–133, 135
  t-cell reduction under, 138
  test, 140–141
  triglyceride levels, 138
  vitamin B6 depletion, 143–144
  zinc depletion, 143–144
Sugar
  addiction, 181–182
  effects of, 182–184
  eliminating from diet, 181–185
  and osteoporosis, 120
Sulfa drugs, and ascorbic acid, 83–84
Sulfonamides, and gastrointestinal absorption, 85
Sulfur, in wound healing, 102
Sulpha Salazine, 80
Supplements
  basic formula for, 95
  for hospital patients, 93–94
  for optimal nutrition, 93
Surfactants
  and cholesterol, 82
  and vitamin A, 82
Sympathetic nervous system, reaction to stress, 132–133, 135
Synergism, 7

T-cells, and stress, 138
Tetracycline
  and calcium, 85
  and fat-soluble vitamins, 82
Thalidomide, 86
Thiamin, 15–16
  and baking soda, 70
Thyroid hormones, and vitamin E, 83

216   Index

Tofu, 119–120
Toxins, and antioxidants, 112
Trace elements, 96
Triglycerides
  and carnitine, 114
  and stress, 138
Tryptophan, as serotonin precursor, 143
Tween, 80, 82
Tyramine, and monoamine oxidase inhibitors, 87
Tyrosine, and phenylalanine, 1

Utilization, 71

Vanadium, 41–42
Vegetables, and dietary antigens, 72
Vitamin(s), 3
  A, 9–10, 82
  B-complex, 4, 5, 70, 184
  bioflavonoids, 14–15
  biotin, 23
  C, 4–5, 13–14, 68, 70, 79, 81, 83, 88, 96, 108, 110, 114, 121–122, 123, 142–143. *See also* Ascorbic acid
  as catalyst, 3
  choline, 25–26
  cobalamin (B12), 20–21, 84
  D, 10–11, 79, 82, 83, 88
  deficiencies, 50–51, 91
  drug interactions, 79–87
  E, 11–12, 79, 83, 102–103, 110, 114, 146
  and enzymes, 3–4
  fat-soluble, 5–6, 82
  folic acid, 22
  inositol, 24
  K, 12–13, 79, 80, 82, 87
  metabolism, 3
  niacin (B3), 17–18
  PABA, 25
  pantothenic acid (B5), 18–19
  pyridoxine (B6), 19–20, 84, 183
  riboflavin (B2), 16–17
  thiamin (B1), 15–16, 68
  water-soluble, 4–5, 82, 83

Warfarin, absorption, 85
Water
  contaminated, 53
  and sodium, 87
Weight loss, and cancer, 111
Wheat, 177, 180
Wheat flour, refining process, 66
Wheat protein, as dietary antigen, 72
Whirlpool therapy, 102
Wholistic therapy, 107–108
Women, and health care, 127–128

Yogurt, "live," 101, 195

Zinc, 33–34
  and cadmium, 112
  and cancer, 110
  and collagen, 102
  stress and depletion of, 143–144